Bearing Witness

LIFE WRITING SERIES

In the **Life Writing Series**, Wilfrid Laurier University Press publishes life writing and new life-writing criticism and theory in order to promote autobiographical accounts, diaries, letters, and testimonials written and/or told by women and men whose political, literary, or philosophical purposes are central to their lives. The Series features accounts written in English, or translated into English from French or the languages of the First Nations, or any of the languages of immigration to Canada.

From its inception, **Life Writing** has aimed to foreground the stories of those who may never have imagined themselves as writers or as people with lives worthy of being (re)told. Its readership has expanded to include scholars, youth, and avid general readers both in Canada and abroad. The Series hopes to continue its work as a leading publisher of life writing of all kinds, as an imprint that aims for both broad representation and scholarly excellence, and as a tool for both historical and autobiographical research.

As its mandate stipulates, the Series privileges those individuals and communities whose stories may not, under normal circumstances, find a welcoming home with a publisher. **Life Writing** also publishes original theoretical investigations about life writing, as long as they are not limited to one author or text.

Series Editor
Marlene Kadar
Humanities Division, York University

Manuscripts to be sent to
Lisa Quinn, Acquisitions Editor
Wilfrid Laurier University Press
75 University Avenue West
Waterloo, Ontario, Canada N2L 3C5

We acknowledge the support of the Canada Council for the Arts for our publishing program. We acknowledge the financial support of the Government of Canada through the Book Publishing Industry Development Program for our publishing activities.

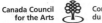 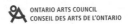

Library and Archives Canada Cataloguing in Publication

Bearing witness : living with ovarian cancer / edited by Kathryn Carter and Laurie Elit.

(Life writing series)
Includes bibliographical references.
Issued also in electronic format.
ISBN 978-1-55458-055-2

1. Ovaries—Cancer—Patients—Canada—Biography. I. Carter, Kathryn, 1966– II. Elit, Laurie III. Life writing series

RC280.O8B43 2009   362.1'969946500922   C2009-903700-9

Library and Archives Canada Cataloguing in Publication

Bearing witness [electronic resource] : living with ovarian cancer / edited by Kathryn Carter and Laurie Elit.

(Life writing series)
Includes bibliographical references.
Electronic edited collection in PDF, ePub, and XML formats. Issued also in print format.
ISBN 978-1-55458-163-4

1. Ovaries—Cancer—Patients—Canada—Biography. I. Carter, Kathryn, 1966– II. Elit, Laurie III. Life writing series

RC280.O8B43 2009   362.1'969946500922

Cover design by Sandra Friesen. Text design by C. Bonas-Taylor.

© 2009 Wilfrid Laurier University Press
Waterloo, Ontario, Canada
www.wlupress.wlu.ca

This book is printed on FSC recycled paper and is certified Ecologo. It is made from 100% post-consumer fibre, processed chlorine free, and manufactured using biogas energy.

Printed in Canada

Bearing Witness
Stories of Women Living
with Ovarian Cancer

Kathryn Carter and Laurie Elit,
editors

Wilfrid Laurier University Press

Contents

Acknowledgments

The authors would like to thank those who were instrumental in creating the manuscript and seeing it through to publication. Kathryn Carter and Geraldine Lavery interviewed the women whose stories make up this book, though Geraldine Lavery did most of the interviews. The names of the women we interviewed have been changed to protect their privacy. We have tried to remove the names of all health care staff and references to the locations where care was delivered. Carolyn Usher transcribed the taped interviews into raw written material. Kathryn edited and reshaped some of the stories, and Thom Froese took the raw and half-edited material to create these finished stories. Ethics approval for this work was obtained from the McMaster University Ethics Review Board on February 28, 2002. The editors would also like to acknowledge a grant from Wilfrid Laurier University that allowed Gerry Lavery to prepare the bibliography on illness and narrativity that appears at the end of this book. A special thank you goes to the nursing staff at the Hamilton Regional Cancer Centre who shared this project with many women who had ovarian cancer. It's those women who have shared their stories here. To them we owe our greatest debt of gratitude.

Proceeds of this book will go toward research endeavours in ovarian cancer via the National Ovarian Cancer Association
#101–145 Front Street East
Toronto, Ontario M5A 1E3
Phone: 1-877-413-7970
www.ovariancanada.org

This book has been made possible in part through an educational grant from Schering Canada, Inc. Pointe-Claire, Quebec

Introduction

by Dr. Laurie Elit,
Gynecologic Oncologist

Personal stories are ... easier to relate to than principles and people love to hear them. They capture our attention and we remember them longer.

—Rick Warren, The Purpose Driven Life

PERSONAL STORIES MAY BE EASIER to remember, as Rick Warren says above, but this does not mean they are always easy to hear or easy to read. What you are about to read is, I admit, difficult. It is a collection of stories that have been created from interviews with women living with recurrent ovarian cancer. The goal of this project was to create a book, unlike any that currently exist, about women's experiences of ovarian cancer with an approach that recognizes terminal cancer as not simply a medical event but a personal trauma. Currently, few books attempt to address the lived experience of ovarian cancer, and those that do focus on single cases. This book presents the stories of several women; however, the interviews with these women were not generated with any specific set of questions. You will notice that the stories don't follow any particular plot or pattern because the discussions about the women's illnesses and their lives developed organically. The collected stories that follow contribute to ongoing scholarly discussions about life writing and trauma, and they will also provide a springboard for further qualitative investigations that may lead to better communication between patients and health care providers as they manage this deadly disease. Perhaps most importantly, and I know that I value the book for this reason, the stories will be useful to those reflecting on the meaning of cancer in their own lives. When I think of the women I care for, I have wished very much that they had a resource such as this book.

The women who were interviewed for this book were at various stages in their journeys with recurrent ovarian cancer. They were under the care of the Juravanski Cancer Centre in Hamilton, Ontario, which services 2.5 million residents in the Hamilton, Niagara, Haldimand, and Brant Local Health Integrated Network. In order to participate, the women could be of any age with a diagnosis of recurrent ovarian cancer. Women were excluded if they were unable to converse in English; if they had health problems such as deafness, mental illness, or addictive disorders that altered understanding or made communication difficult; or if they did not provide consent.

Ovarian cancer affects 1 in 70 women. Some call it the disease that whispers. Many cancers, if found early, are curable. This is also true for ovarian cancer. The problem is that the symptoms of this disease are so vague (bloating, changes in bowel habits, flatulence, back pain, pelvic discomfort) that they could be the result of many nonserious conditions. Many women are diagnosed only once the disease has spread widely throughout the abdominal cavity. They often present to the physician with a large, distended abdomen full of fluid, which we refer to as ascites.

The treatment for ovarian cancer is aggressive surgery to determine how widespread the disease is and to try to remove as much tumour as possible. This is followed by chemotherapy. Upon finishing these two treatment modalities the patient is followed regularly. If after five years the disease has not come back, it is considered cured. If the disease comes back, the chances of cure are extremely small. The health care staff can try to improve symptoms through additional cycles of chemotherapy; however, ovarian cancer has a pattern of continual recurrence. Unfortunately, the cancer eventually develops resistance to the drugs that are used, and in time, they stop working.

Treatment decision making during the course of ovarian cancer can be stressful for patients and families. Health care providers have practice guidelines or algorithms that distill the many, many research studies and offer principles that can be applied to each circumstance. For example, doctors need to assess whether surgery or initial chemotherapy is the best approach when a woman first presents with a pelvic mass. And when and if the disease recurs, the doctor needs to evaluate the available research to determine which chemotherapy drugs will be most useful. However, at the same time, the patient and her family are in a very different emotional space. At the first clinical visit, they will be digesting bad news about the cancer being active and hearing recommendations from the health care team. Often they are presented with information about side effects and outcomes. A lot is said at these first meetings, and the information can be overwhelming. Patients have to decide whether to accept treatment or not, and sometimes they have more than two options to consider. If a woman is having trouble assimilating the information, the wisest course of action may be to take time out. A woman may want to walk away and reflect on the verbal and written information; she may want to do her own homework. Part of this homework may include setting priorities and goals: the woman might ask herself what she imagines as the most positive outcome of her cancer and then try to discern if her doctor offers her a chance of getting there. Talking with a team nurse or having a more in-depth conversation with a social worker may help the woman sort through and identify her priorities. Speaking with other health care providers (like a family doctor), searching the Internet, or getting a second opinion are things a woman can do to better understand what is happening to her. She can then come back to her health care team with clear goals and questions that will improve her journey, as well as her satisfaction with her decision and the health care path she chooses to follow. My research on women's perceptions about treatment decision making for ovarian cancer found that at the early stages, women found friends and family members who advocated for them in a positive way most helpful. Another tool that will be helpful to women newly diagnosed is a book like this that shows other women's paths, revealing that no two journeys are alike.

Those of us who are physically well may look at these stories and see only bleakness. I am always humbled when I am reminded that the woman with ovarian cancer is a woman first. The following stories work to remind us that a woman was living her life when ovarian cancer came to co-exist with her for a time. She has a past, a character that has been developed over the years, and she brings these things into her journey with the disease. These coping skills and inner fortitude will shine through as she learns to deal with the physical discomforts of the disease and the emotional shadow of knowing that her life will be cut short. Tonight, however, as darkness falls, this physician sits and the tears just keep coming. It has been a particularly hard week. Three women in my practice have died of ovarian cancer. Aside from sharing a common disease, what connected all these women? Well, they were in their mid-50s; they were all my patients; but most importantly, all exemplified the spirit that I hope we have captured in the stories you are about to read. As a physician, I have the privilege of walking alongside women during their journeys through ovarian cancer. Some of these women react to their circumstances with anger, frustration, and despair. However, other women, like these three, cause my staff and me to stand in the wings feeling proud to have known them. We take comfort in their courage. We are amazed by their gentleness. They possess a way of making others feel blessed by spending time in their presence.

Several years ago, as I worked through my master's thesis, "Patient Preference for Treatment Decision Making in Advanced Ovarian Cancer," I saw that there were two groups of women. Some looked at their circumstances as if the cup were half empty—woe is me, look at what I have lost. This is certainly a very understandable perspective, given the life-changing impact of ovarian cancer. But then there is another group of women. They look at their ovarian cancer in terms of the cup being half full; they find a place where they are thankful for all that is in their lives, especially for the people who surround them. As we share a glimpse into the lives of women who are dealing with recurrent ovarian cancer, it is my prayer for each of you that whether you have ovarian cancer or know someone with this disease, you will catch this spirit. These women have learned to live life, whatever the hardships. I think especially of Esther, who survived Auschwitz in her teen years only to battle with ovarian cancer in her senior years. She was the catalyst in the creation of this collection in that she inspired us to collect and share these stories so that others may be able to see and understand the importance of rising above circumstances. She spoke of her journey in terms of survival, a way of coping that she developed no doubt during those dark days in Poland. All the women in this book show us what they value, and how they evaluate their lives, as they walk through uncertainty one day at a time. Their responses are learned from the lives they have lived; they did not arrive at answers by reading a manual. Their highly individualistic responses are evident in the way they describe relationships and how they narrate experience: in other words, it shows up in shared stories. I will always remember the evening when Kathryn Carter and I sat at the feet of Esther and heard her powerful story. It was the night that this book began.

As a result of my desire to document individualistic responses like Esther's, I began qualitative research based on the guidelines put forward by the *BMJ* (*British Medical Journal*) and *JAMA* (*Journal of the American Medical Association*). It is an approach that focuses on understanding processes, experiences, or socially constructed meanings, and it adopts an insider's perspective. The interview team developed a semi-structured interview guide that explored such issues as how the cancer was diagnosed and the stage of the disease. We asked the women what they saw for their future and what kind of meaning they attributed to this journey with cancer. We tape-recorded and then transcribed the interviews, checking each transcription for accuracy against the original audiotaped interview. After editing the stories, we made them available to the woman or her family for further feedback if necessary.

For the health care professional, what you can learn from these stories is that patients need to be assured that you or your staff will be there whenever things get rough. Many of the women with ovarian cancer were diagnosed after a long period of symptoms, and there is a sense that if things had been caught earlier, the outcome would have been improved. Patients want to be seen as a person with the disease of ovarian cancer, not as the disease only. As you stand in the presence of suffering over time (whether you are a family member caring for a chronically ill loved one or a health care provider who is taking calls and repeating assessments because something keeps going wrong) you realize that small things are important. Maybe it's a smile when you know that the needle hurts, or a joke about an ostomy appliance. Character is tried and tested in small challenges, but it truly shines through when the going gets really rough. Sometimes that means spending time with a patient, sometimes that means remembering to ask about things that are important to them, such as the trip to the cottage or the 50th wedding anniversary celebration. Listening to women's voices in these stories reminds us that they are women and not just patients.

As you prepare to open these pages, do so with a box of tissues.

Esther

[I marched] into hell for a heavenly cause,
And I know if I'll only be true to this glorious quest,
That my heart will lie peaceful and calm
When I'm laid to my rest,
And the world will be better for this.

—"The Impossible Dream," lyrics by Joe Darion,
   from *Man of La Mancha*

She says that she "caught God by the foot" once by surviving Auschwitz. Now she faces the effects of both a stroke and ovarian cancer. But Esther takes it all in stride, and commenting on how much she values her husband and other family members who love her, she simply notes, "I think that I am fortunate. I am grateful for my life."

MY LIFE HAS BEEN EVENTFUL AND I have been very fortunate. I was born in Hungary and still quite young when Nazis invaded my hometown. My family and I were sent to Auschwitz. I was 14 at the time; I was young and strong. I had the job of carting dead bodies away in a wheelbarrow. I lost most of my family, and when I managed to escape death, I felt that I had caught God by the foot.

   After that I returned to Hungary. My husband lived in the next town over and he had lost his family in the camps too, so we married; we were only teenagers. In 1951 we decided to move to Canada for a second chance at life. We were so poor when we arrived. We ate every bit of canned food that we could afford, and we could only guess what was inside by looking at the picture on the front because we couldn't yet speak English. Our first table was just some wooden crates. Eventually I got a job that used my training in chemistry, but I remember trying to come home from that job and spending hours lost on a bus because I couldn't tell where it was going. I arrived home to a very worried husband.

When my husband landed a good job, he treated me like a queen. He insisted that I buy whatever I need for my daughter and myself, even if he did without. Yes, our beautiful daughter arrived in the 1950s. We started buying houses at that time, and we must have moved 12 to 13 times. My husband always bought rundown houses and fixed them up to sell them. I took off more wallpaper than you can ever imagine. The next move that I make will be a different one; I won't take much.

I had a stroke before I knew that I had ovarian cancer. It affected my right arm, and it has been more trouble really than the cancer. I didn't know about the cancer until I realized I was getting stout, so I went to the doctor.

I have no pain with the cancer. I don't know how I would react if I were to have pain. I hope that they have the knowledge today that it shouldn't hurt. I know by my age that I am getting close to the end anyway. Everybody should realize that whatever medical science tries to do to prolong life, if someone is healthy and they try to prolong their life longer for them, it is nice. But if someone is ill and lives with a sickness that will kill them anyway, that isn't good. So I think of the end, because I know that it is coming.

There should be some people who know how to teach people when there is no way out. On a psychological level, I don't think that I would be able to do that; you would have to be an expert to be able to explain to them that it is coming, and one has to prepare themselves. When you get to 75 or 80 years old and you are ill then you know that it is coming. I am not going to be surprised. I asked my family physician and when the time comes I am going to ask my oncologist to help me as much as they can because I don't think that I have a high tolerance for pain. I know that they can't kill me, but they can help to control the pain.

Anyway, I do have a happy life even as I am. I make myself have a happy life. I think that I am fortunate. I am grateful for my life.

EVERY MORNING, MY HUSBAND GETS up at 7 o'clock, and then he makes breakfast. The "Queen of Sheba" (that's me) will come out at 7:30 and have breakfast. When he sees me, he says, "Good morning, gorgeous" every morning! Then someone will come and pick me up to go to the bank—since they took my licence away I have to get a ride. My husband will not be home, so one of my girlfriends will pick me up and take me to the bank. And around 10:30 we will go to the mall, and I am going to buy the best toaster oven there is, one that will last as long as I will. At noon I have to come home because my husband will be home for lunch, and we will have lunch together with whoever is here.

Our routine is pretty set. He goes to the office (he goes in at 8 a.m.); he comes home for lunch every day; he goes in to lie down for an hour; and he comes home after work at 6 for dinner. In the afternoon I watch the soap operas, and if it is not interesting I read a few pages. Later in the afternoon another girlfriend of mine will come—she stays with me until 5. She is going to tell me about the concert that she went to last night. At 5:10, the doctor's wife comes—she comes every day and stays until my husband comes, and then she talks to him for 10 minutes too, and then we have dinner. I don't do the cooking anymore. I have a lady who lives with me, and she does the cooking. And after supper if we are bored we play gin rummy. At 9 p.m. it is bedtime for Bonzo. So that is my typical day.

I want to go to my grandson's bar mitzvah. I told him yesterday. That will be the 22nd of May next year. That's my oldest grandson. I have three grandsons and a beautiful daughter and a son-in-law with a sense of humour. He's always telling me jokes. I have a loving husband. I have been fortunate. This isn't an up or a down in my life; it is an ending. It isn't a very nice exit, but it's an exit.

Esther's family came together for shiva almost four years after her diagnosis of ovarian cancer.

Bev

The woods are lovely, dark and deep.
But I have promises to keep,
And miles to go before I sleep ...

—from "Stopping by the Woods on a Snowy Evening,"
by Robert Frost

As a painter, Bev knew how to see beauty in life. And she knew consistency, having lived in the same house for 42 years. But then her lung collapsed one day while she was attending a painting seminar in the southern United States. And after being rushed back to her hometown via air ambulance, Bev learned her diagnosis: ovarian cancer. At age 62, she would be left to find even more value in her closest relationships and in those precious moments of restoration, at places like the cottage lake.

I HAVE LIVED HERE ALL MY LIFE, in the same house for 42 years with my husband. We raised three daughters. Two of them are now married: one with four kids and one with two kids. This year I didn't have the energy for Christmas shopping, so I let them do their own. Last year we managed. You have to pace yourself.

When I was diagnosed with cancer, I was 62. My sister's oldest boy had been in the former USSR in the army and had developed brain tumours, which they feel now are related to that experience. He passed away a few months before my diagnosis. I was diagnosed early in 2001, and my sister, who is a decade older than me, was diagnosed with breast cancer the day of my first chemo. Our parents had never had cancer, so it was quite a blow for us as a family. There were three children in my family: my sister, my brother, and myself. My sister had a large family and I had three, so they all had to go and be tested for breast and ovarian cancer.

Holidays Down South

It all started in 2001. It was at the start of our holidays. We had gone south. I was going to a three-day painting seminar, and each day it got a little more difficult to move. Even before I left, I had complained to the doctor that I was bloated and uncomfortable, but I got the same old response: "You're an old lady. Take the weight off. Yada yada." So anyway, we got down south and I managed to finish the seminar, and the next morning my husband took me to the clinic that was right across from the hospital. They took me for an X-ray and immediately said, "You are going across the road to the hospital." When I said we could get home in two days, the nurse said, "You don't have two days. Your lung has collapsed."

So we went to the hospital. They admitted me, put a needle in my back, and drained off two litres of fluid. It was up between the lung and the lining of the lung. That was a Monday, and when they examined the fluid they found it was full of malignant cells. When they did the CT scans and whatnot they found ovarian cancer that had already spread and was in the later stages. They drained another two litres on the Friday and put me on an air ambulance back to my hometown on the Saturday. The thoracic surgeon put a permanent drain in my side and drained the rest of the fluid and then blew in some talc to cement the liner to the lung, so the fluid couldn't get back up. He arranged for us to meet the gynecological oncologist at the cancer centre three weeks later.

The gynecologic oncologist said that I would have to have a complete hysterectomy, but first she wanted me to have two bouts of chemotherapy using Taxol and platin, I think, before the operation to try to shrink the tumours. I started the chemo early in April, went through the two sessions, and then had the operation later in the spring.

It was kind of like Murphy's Law, because whatever could go wrong did go wrong. Thankfully, the operation went well. They were able to remove the omentum, which is the fatty layer that goes over the abdomen. It was wrapped around the upper bowel. The omentum itself was full of cancer, and they were able to remove that without going into the bowel. And they scraped away as much tumour as they could, and felt that the following chemotherapy would take care of the rest.

But when I was in the hospital I got pneumonia after a couple of days, and then after the pneumonia all my electrolytes went kerfluey, so I ended up staying in the hospital eleven days rather than five or six. The following chemotherapy did miraculously take care of the tumours, because when I had another CT scan at the end of the summer, there were no tumours showing. They had gone away.

I went for a CT scan and then went to see the oncologist at the end of January. The CT scan showed that the cancer was back with a vengeance, and it was in the lymph glands in the groin, in the spleen, and in the lining of the diaphragm, and there was a thickening of the wall of the lung, stomach, and the aorta. So it had really taken over. The oncologist said it wasn't necessary to start another chemotherapy right then; we could wait until the point when I was so uncomfortable that I was looking forward to it. I think that she felt that starting it in two or three months wasn't really going to matter.

More Treatments

We went to the West Coast for a little holiday, and I ended up in hospital overnight with quite severe pain in my back. The doctor there recommended that we head home. This was over Easter, so when I saw my oncologist after the Easter week she started me on chemo that day. That session of chemo was really rough. It was fed intravenously five days a week for an hour, and then I was to be off two weeks and start again. But it was so hard on my system that they put it off for three weeks in between.

At first I seemed to be doing all right, so we thought we would head to the cottage on the Friday after my last treatment in early May. We thought we'd stay there for the summer and just come back for the chemo. But that first weekend, I ended up in the hospital because they couldn't stop me from throwing up. The anti-nausea drugs weren't working on me, even though they were administering them intravenously. Then I got over that.

After the next treatment in June, I had the first day's dosage and everything was fine until 9 o'clock that night. All of sudden I started vomiting nonstop, so I ended up back in my local hospital for a week. Then they arranged for me to have home care when I got home. They kept me on intravenous all day and all night, and then they would unhook me to go back for chemo in the morning. Then they would come back and administer the anti-nausea drugs. As fast as they poured them in my arm, I was spewing them out.

August was the last session of chemo, and it was like a miracle happened because I didn't have any reaction from it at all! It was crazy. My husband and I would look at each other in the TV room and say, "Okay, when's it going to hit?" When we asked the oncologist later, she said that every drug and treatment is different. Every person is different, and if you have six sessions of it, every session could be different for each person.

I had a CT in September and I saw my oncologist a week later. She said it was the same. There was no change. The tumours hadn't grown, but they hadn't shrunk either. At this point the doctor said that I could either go on and take VP16 or some other chemo drug or be part of a clinical trial that was showing a lot of promise. The trials are done on advanced cancers that aren't responding to any other treatments. It is a live chicken virus called Newcastle chicken virus, and it is administered intravenously.

The first one is administered over a 3-hour time period, and I will be monitored at the hospital for 24 hours. This will start a week from today, and then the following dosages are given over an hour at the cancer centre, with an hour for observation. This provirus, they tell you right off that for the first 10 days you will feel that you have the worst flu of your life with fever, chills, nausea, vomiting, and diarrhea. You name it, you are going to get it.

The thing is that I don't like the alternative. I just have to keep on trying, and this provirus seems to be having remarkable results. They are very excited about it. I think that this is the first ovarian cancer that they have used it on, but I could be wrong. Mostly they have been working with other types of cancer. It is a virus that only attacks the cancer cells, not the normal cells. The cancerous ones get kind of red and angry and swollen. With your abdomen it's okay because there is room for swelling, but I had to go for a CT scan for the abdomen and chest and also one on my head, because even though there is no indication of a brain tumour, even the smallest one could be deadly if it was to swell. So they are very careful about all the tests that they give. There is no alternative.

Living for Family

My youngest grandchildren just turned three and four this week. Last spring when they pulled up to the cottage they saw me with no hair for the first time. The littlest one, who was three at the time, said, "Grandma, where is your hair?" And she was quite shocked by it. But then this last time that I was in the hospital, my daughter brought the two little ones in to see me and they were really good, which is amazing because they are just full of beans. And when I came home from the hospital she was there that day at the cottage. She said, "Grandma, you don't have to go to the hospital again?" and I said, "No." She said, "Oh, that's good. Grandma, you are all better now."

They know that I have been sick, but we don't harp on it. Particularly this summer, when the chemo took a lot out of me, it was easy to tell that I didn't have much energy. My other grandchildren are in their teens, and they are aware of what is going on. They seem to be dealing with it well, and they are good with me. They just act normally. They all seem to cope with it, and we joke about the lack of hair. My daughter wrote this wonderful letter to me:

Dear Mom,

   This has been a tough year, and I can't even imagine what it has been like for you. You have been amazing. You never complained and you never let us know how bad you really feel. I only hope that if I ever have to face something like this that I can do it with half the grace and dignity that you have shown. You are my angel of courage and I love you.

   Terry

There are certainly days that I get down and get tired of feeling lousy. My husband has been such a help, and I could have never gotten through without him. I pray and I have my holy waters. I just have to keep going because I don't like the alternative. Also, I painted this past summer quite a bit. I taught painting for nine years, and my students also take good care of me. They call, and they are on the Internet. They are all really swell women, and they are all more than supportive of me. So I have had wonderful support. Last year from February through the past Christmas, there has not been a day gone by when the postman didn't bring a card. It was wonderful. People don't realize just how much impact a card has.

Our cottage up north also really lifts my spirits, and it has for years. We are a block away from the water, but we are on a beautiful park that is on the water. It is just so restorative up there. I know when my cousin would do hands-on meditation, and they asked you to think of yourself in a peaceful setting, I always think of myself sitting on the shore at the lake. It's a wonderful place. This summer I had a PICC line inserted in my arm for my intravenous, and I couldn't go in the water because I couldn't get it wet, and so I would go in up to my waist and then my husband would hold my hands and I would kind of dunk down. Then in the fall it clogged up, so luckily I had to have it out and I could go swimming again! It was wonderful to dive down under the water when you have just kind of been bouncing around in it all summer, so that was good. I was glad to get rid of it for a few weeks.

If I spoke to another woman with ovarian cancer, I would say, "Just try to keep your spirits up. And don't let anybody tell you that you are finished." When I was down south I was told that my cancer was very advanced and that there really probably wasn't anything that could be done for it. But when somebody says that to you, you have nowhere to go but up. You just have to keep on going. I remember when my nephew was sick with the brain tumour, he was going to try a new treatment, and my sister said to me, "I don't know why he is going to put himself through the pain and the agony of it." And I said, "When you want to live, you just do it."

Bev's family celebrated her life 22 months after her diagnosis of ovarian cancer.

Lisa

It has been said that our world is shaped by the stories we tell;
and likewise, we as individuals are sculpted by the stories we hear.

—Christopher Coppernoll, *Secrets of a Faith Well Lived*

Lisa was the model of good health. She took care of herself through a disciplined life of exercise and good eating. A neonatal nurse, she also loved to be on top of her work game. But when her life of order came crashing down with her diagnosis of ovarian cancer, she was forced to re-evaluate what was left. Knowing that knowledge is power, she decided she would talk to her teenage daughter about it all as openly as possible, and spare her the type of pain that Lisa herself felt as a girl when her own mother had the fatal sickness.

I HAVE ONE DAUGHTER, AND I would like her to know later on down the line when she picks up this book that it was me in this discussion. I am 45 and I will be 46 in September. I was diagnosed when I had just turned 40. So it's been a little over five years.

I had been feeling unwell for about three to six months, just general tiredness. I weighed about 103 pounds. I was a runner and I used to eat phenomenal meals and still stayed that weight. I was extremely active—I did kayaking and running—and I had an eight-year-old daughter and a full-time job. In the last 20 years of work, I think that I might have called in sick maybe twice. And at that time, I had called in sick three times in as many months, and actually my husband brought that to my attention.

He said, "Are you sure that you are all right? Maybe you should go and see a doctor."

I said, "No, no, it's really nothing."

This was because the symptoms that I was having were just so general that I didn't really feel anything. I was just really tired all the time, and I would get irritated very quickly and didn't have as much patience as I had had in the past. Just little things bugged me. I never sweat the little things, just the big stuff.

Anyway, I was out running one morning, my daughter and I, and I bent down to tie my shoe, and my knee came up into my abdomen and I felt very full. That was pretty much all I felt, and as soon as I felt that I didn't go for a run. I went home and lay down and had a good poke around at my belly, and I could feel a golf ball–sized lump to the left of my belly button. I was very thin and in very good shape, and you could almost see it when I was lying flat.

So I made an appointment with the gynecologist and went and she was absolutely wonderful. I went for the appointment in the morning. I went for the ultrasound in the afternoon, and they told me right away they saw it. It was eight inches long and six inches wide, and he figured it weighed about eight pounds. It went from my right ovary and down underneath my uterus and came back up, and I was feeling the tip of it, which had come back up one side of my uterus. And that's how we found it. He told me right away.

I said, "Well, why don't we do a biopsy right away?"

And they said no. They didn't want to do that at that point because they risked the possibility of leaving a little opening and the cells coming out to the abdomen.

So I went in and had surgery, and sure enough it weighed close to eight pounds. It was just like I was pregnant. I waited three weeks for surgery, maybe a month, and by then I had gained 18 pounds and it was all fluid. I looked like I was six months pregnant. In fact, when I went into surgery, it was day surgery, and one of the ladies sitting next to me said, "Oh, do you know what you are going to have?"

And trying not to embarrass her, I said, "Well, I am pretty sure what I am going to have."

And she said, "Oh, will it be a boy or a girl?"

I said, "Well, actually it is a tumour that has been growing for a while."

She was horrified and I tried to console her. I said, "It's okay, don't worry. You never knew."

Then, two weeks later, after I recovered from the surgery, I had Taxol and carboplatin treatments for about five months, six full cycles. Then by

July it had grown back (my surgery was in May), and it attached itself to a blood vessel that was in my abdomen.

So, I went to the cancer centre and there was a fellow there who dealt with aggressive surgery. I had already had two cycles of chemotherapy and then had to have the tumour removed because they were afraid that it was going to grow even further. I was extremely sick. I lost a lot of blood. I don't remember very much. Most of what I am telling you about the second surgery is from what my husband has told me. I spent a couple of weeks in ICU and got lots of rounds of blood, and I recovered, as stubborn as I am. In some of my follow-up visits, the doctor said that if I wasn't quite as fit as I was, I probably wouldn't have made it through. So I was really pretty lucky.

I thought that it was all just part of my life, but now in retrospect I was pretty darn lucky—someone was watching over me. When you tell the story to people they are just amazed and in awe. And to me it is just one of those things. You know, lots of families have diabetes and heart disease, and our family just happens to have cancer. My sister was 35 years old and my mom was 35 years old when she was diagnosed with breast cancer. She had a mastectomy, and 13 years later, she had her second mastectomy because it had returned. Then my sister.

When I was 35, I was sure that one of us was going to get it, because my mom's mom also had "female cancer." At that point in time they didn't exactly say what it was, but it was some sort of female problem. I had assumed it was something to do with the ovaries or uterus. She died at 52, and then my mom was 62 when she died, and my sister was diagnosed with breast cancer at 35. She had a terrible time trying to get it diagnosed. They kept saying that she was only 35 and there was no way that it could be cancer. They took multiple mammograms, and she had a mammogram every month for five months and it was nonspecific. Finally, she pushed for a biopsy, and sure enough by then it had spread and it was in her lymph nodes and had gone into her stomach and into her bowels. She had a colostomy, and it wasn't a year later that she died. She was 36 and she left me too.

She left behind a daughter, 13, and a son who was 14, and it was extremely difficult for them. And so every woman in the family on my mom's side has had cancer. Her sister died of a brain tumour behind the eyes. Plus there was her mom, my mom, my sister, and now me. I have one niece (my sister's daughter) and my daughter. And this is why I am telling my story.

Anyway, when I went to the doctor's office she thought that I was pregnant right away. She asked me when my last menstrual period was, and I had had my tubes tied after my daughter was born and had just finished my cycle, so I knew that I could not be pregnant. My daughter was eight, so it had been eight years since I had my tubes tied. We did a pregnancy test anyway, but on the exam she realized that it was something more. She did a pelvic and internal exam and realized right away that I wasn't pregnant. There was no placenta and the uterus hadn't expanded. In fact, it had decreased in size due to the tumour invading from behind. She also tested my thyroid. She thought it might be thyroid because I was just tired, and that was the only symptom I had—I was just very tired and listless.

Since being diagnosed I have talked to a lot of friends of mine who have minor aches and complaints, and my advice to them is to go and check it out, you just never know. When I called the doctor about my problem, they said the flu was going around. Or they check your eyes, ears, nose, and throat. But try to get someone to really listen to you that it goes deeper than just being tired. It's important that you know your body best. I can't emphasize that enough. It is always so easy for other people to negate the way that you are feeling and to bring up suggestions for why you are feeling that way, which is perfectly normal.

Friends do it all the time and they don't mean any harm by it; they are just trying to help you and give you some sort of validation. You know there is flu going around and so and so was sick last week. That's trying to validate how you are feeling. But really, in doing that, it delays your response to your symptoms, and you don't go and check it out because it might just be a virus and that kind of thing. So we tend not to jump on it right away. With our kids, we are always in the emergency room for one thing or another, but not when it comes to us.

I am a neonatal intensive care nurse. I have been for the last 20 years, and I absolutely love it: the high stress, the intensive situations, recognizing symptom change from one minute to the next minute with those tiny, premature babies who can't tell you anything. I love being on top of symptoms and on top of condition changes. And it took me three months of being tired to go and do something about it. I had every excuse in the book. I thought, I am just constipated, or I haven't been running quite as much, or maybe I need to take a multivitamin, or I didn't get a full serving of vegetables this week. You know, all of those kinds of things. And you are just generally too busy—your husband needs this, your child needs this, and your neighbour calls you, and you need to go to soccer practice. Whatever it is, there is always something. The dryer's broken or the plumbing is leaking in the basement. There is always something that is going to go on day to day, so you just ignore the things that aren't screaming at you.

Until you find a lump or something else, and then of course by then it's too late. I mean who knows … maybe if I had gone to the doctor sooner. Of course, you can't "should've" yourself to death. But I should have gone right away when I felt tired and listless and knew that I wasn't quite myself. When I had found the lump before I went to see the doctor, I told my husband about it, and when I was lying down on the bed, I was doing an abdominal quadrant feel, going from quadrant to quadrant. I knew that cancer ran in my family, but I was looking for breast cancer. I taught my daughter from when she was little how to look for little lumps in her torso, and I knew right away that it was ovarian cancer. I don't know whether that was any medical training. It was almost instinctive.

I sat with my husband on the couch and I told him that I had found a lump, and he said, "Did you make an appointment with the doctor?"

I said to him, "I am really sorry, but I believe that I have ovarian cancer."

And the two of us sat and wept for what seemed like hours. Then when I went to the doctor and was diagnosed, and I came home and confirmed the diagnosis to him. He just stood and looked at me, and I started to cry because there was a confirmation there.

And I said to him, "You don't seem as upset."

And he said, "No. I cried before when you told me, and I knew that you knew what you were talking about, and I knew you had it. So it was just a confirmation for you."

It was the funniest interaction; it was very different. And my husband has been so supportive. I was absolutely blessed in being paired up with him. God absolutely knew what he was doing. We have been together for 18 years. We actually separated and got divorced after 6 years. It was cited as irreconcilable differences, but it was just that we were young and stupid. Then we got back together. We were divorced for 3 years, but we still saw each other and went out. We just lived separately.

When we got back together we got remarried, and now we are older, wiser, more mature, more understanding of each other, less selfish. He has been phenomenal. He is an absolute godsend. I sat next to people in chemotherapy when I was getting IV chemotherapy, and these women would say that they had to run home and make dinner for their kids and their husband and whatever, and I never had to do anything like that. My husband did all the cooking, cleaning, washing, drying, laundry, vacuuming—he did everything, plus he went to work, and I just had to recuperate. He was phenomenal.

My daughter has grown up with it. When my sister passed away, we talked quite a bit about it, and she even knew what cancer was before that. She knew that Nana had breast cancer. My mom was not quite as open. She had breast cancer when she was 35 and we were very young. We were 6 and 2 years old. And she never really talked an awful lot about it, and she certainly would never joke about it. She would never make light of any situation.

When we talked about it, it was very sombre and very serious. My sister and I, when we grew up, made a pact with each other that if and when it happened to us, we wouldn't be like that—we would make sure that everybody knew; we would get as educated as possible. Ignoring it doesn't make it go away. Our kids are going to know about it. They are going to know from when they are little tots that this is what cancer is and that it runs in the family, and it's part of our everyday life like diabetes would be or heart disease or whatever, and that's the way we dealt with it. Open, honest education. Knowledge is power. Open discussions all the time about it—if there are any questions, don't hesitate to ask; don't ever hesitate to look something up or bring something up.

A friend of mine once said to me, "You know, I want to ask you some questions about it, but I am afraid that if I bring it up, you will remember that you have it. It will remind you of having the disease."

I said to her, "There is not a chance that you could ever forget. You can't. It's a part of your life, so don't ever feel that you could ever bring something to my attention that I wasn't already thinking of."

In fact, my husband said, "Don't flatter yourself so much that you could possibly make her think of something that she is not."

So she said, "Okay, I will ask you anything."

Yes, ask anything you can possibly think of. Don't try to push something into the background just because you are afraid of asking. My thought is that what if she didn't ask those questions and a friend of hers was diagnosed with ovarian cancer, and the friend asked her, "Don't you have a friend with ovarian cancer? Does she ever have...?" And she doesn't have the knowledge to answer her friend's question. If she had asked, we could have discussed it, and she could have taken that knowledge that she gained from me and passed it on to someone else.

I think this is what the younger generation believes, but the older, more mature people who are being diagnosed still have another frame of mind because that's their reference point. That's where they grew up from. My father-in-law had a brain tumour, and he just passed this last March. He had it for about two years, and my husband's mom always wanted me to go to the appointments and to ask the questions to the physician and be there. But when we discussed it as a family, she did not want me to do that. My husband comes from a family where his mother never worked. His father was a full-time truck driver and his mother raised nine kids. They are from a little town in northern Ontario, and their attitude was that of years gone by when we really never talked.

We would never even refer to the brain tumour as being cancer. And when I openly said in a discussion that cancer grows, she put her hand up and stopped me and said, "It's not cancer, it's a brain tumour."

I said, "Well, if you would like me to refer to it as a brain tumour, I will do so."

I did that out of respect for them. Nobody else in the family called it cancer either, but still it grew from his frontal lobe down to his spinal cord. My father-in-law died peacefully, after he ended up in a nursing home for the last three weeks. All the family was there. And still to this day they don't talk about it as being cancer.

My daughter talks to me openly about it all. In fact, last year she had a student in her class whose aunt had just been diagnosed with cancer. He was telling his classmates that she was going to lose all of her hair, and he said, "Your mom lost all her hair, didn't she?" She said yes, but she was quick to tell him that it's the treatment that makes them lose their hair, and he was under the impression that it was the cancer that made them lose their hair. And she came home and said, "That is right, isn't it Mom? It's the medicine that you take that makes you bald, it's not the actual cancer." I said, "Yes, you are right."

And after that her teacher had her do a minimal presentation about cancer and about her experience and what cancer is. She said that cancer is normal cells in the body that just started growing abnormally, that you don't lose your hair over it, that you have chemotherapy, and some makes you lose your hair. She said, "My mom had one chemotherapy treatment that didn't make her lose her hair," and they said, "Can't everybody have chemotherapy that doesn't make you lose your hair?" And she said, "That depends on what kind of cancer you have." The teacher later on said that it was wonderful—she was very knowledgeable and sounded like she was authoritative.

The entire exercise validated her knowledge. I have often thought because of some of the questions she has asked, was it a good idea that my sister and I made that pact to give them so much information at such a young age? But based on that, it made me feel validated on the decision that I made years ago. I felt very comfortable, and she said that she wasn't uncomfortable talking to the class about it. She said that there were some classmates' questions that she didn't know the answers to. She said, "I told them I don't know but you can ask your mom's doctor when you go with her, or you can ask your aunt's doctor when you go with her or whoever you go with."

I don't give my daughter any information that she isn't ready to take in. Of course, now she is 14 and she is extremely open about it, and some nights she sits up with me and we have a little cry and she asks, "Are you going to die?" I say, "Not today, I am not going to die today." That's all I can say, and that's what's important.

It's harder when you take the chemotherapy and you don't look well and you are throwing up and you feel tired and you spend quite a bit of time sleeping. That's the time when she feels that the cancer is up front. When we are in between the times, when I am not taking chemotherapy, we take walks together. I don't run anymore; we kayak together and do things like that. And those times put it in the back of her mind that I'm not so sick anymore, and it gives her distance and a reprieve from those feelings.

After I was first diagnosed, I was absolutely overwhelmed by statistics and the feeling that 70 percent of women die within two years, and the other 30 percent die within four years, and that it's exceptional to find someone who lived more than five years. My part of the coping mechanism that we used was knowledge and communication, using the right terminology so it wasn't foreign.

Both my parents were from Britain; they came over after they got married. Both my sister and I were born in Canada. So it was always the four of us: my parents, my sister, and me. When my mom died, my dad buried my mom. When my sister died, he also buried her. As soon as I realized the statistics—I mean, my dad is only 74 and he has a long bloodline, his family lives into their 80s and 90s—I thought there is not a chance in hell that I am going to let my dad bury me! And from then on, that has been a huge part of the attitude that I have about beating this.

That, plus humour, laughing about it, even the open, honest communication about it, you have the opportunity to lighten the situation. Don't miss that opportunity—jump in and make it light because then people who are sitting around feel that this isn't such a horrible thing that they can no longer talk about. You know that if you don't laugh about it, you are just going to sit and sob about it all the time. That's no way to be. And that kind of attitude brings down your emotions and your hopes. It brings you down.

If you're not uplifted all the time and you don't take it on like it is one of life's challenges, then how you deal with it is going to make or break the situation. If you are always sad about it, it's like your body dies when you are diagnosed and they bury you 10 years later. I don't want my husband or my daughter to look back on it and think of having cancer the way that I think about my mom and how quiet we had to be and how we never talked about her. I want to completely live until the day that I can't any longer.

Lisa journeyed for more than five years with ovarian cancer.

Mary

There are two ways to live your life, .
One is as though nothing is a miracle,
The other is as though everything is a miracle.

—Albert Einstein

With nine nieces and nephews, Mary says she was cured of any desire to have any of her own children. Still, it was a shock when at just 37, she was diagnosed with ovarian cancer. She believes it could have been treated sooner, had her family physician responded better to her symptoms. But rather than let anger get the better of her, Mary, along with supportive friends and family, learned to respond to the deadly condition with a unique style of humour and realism.

MY JOURNEY WITH OVARIAN CANCER all started with what appeared to be just a problem with my legs and some breathing problems. They thought I had asthma. My family doctor sent me down to the hospital to get an asthma treatment, and when I got down there, they discovered that I had fluid around my left lung and that caused a cough. They drained the fluid and they said the cough would go away, but it never did; five months later I still had the cough and was still seeing the breathing doctor. I thought, if he can't find the reason why, then I will just have it all my life.

Part of the reason that I was seeing my family doctor was because I was on water pills. I got these because my fingers were swelling up and acting odd and my mother had the same thing. The two-week medication worked for me; everything got smaller but my stomach. My chest, arms, legs got smaller, everything except my stomach. So when I went back to my family doctor, she said, "Here's a one-year prescription, and the longer you are on it the faster it works."

I said "Okay, fine."

Pregnant?!

Then she sent me to see my breathing doctor because I also walked into that office and said, "It has been five months and I still have this cough." I live at home, and my mother sleeps across the hall. She was so exhausted because I was keeping her up at night. So I went and had the interview with the breathing doctor, and he asked me all sorts of questions, including, "When are you expecting?"

I told him, "I'm not!"

I told him about the water pills and that everything had gotten smaller. When he heard that I hadn't had any other tests and that my family doctor hadn't done anything about my stomach not getting smaller, he apparently wrote a rather nasty note to her wanting to know why she hadn't taken one look at my stomach and the results of the water pills and asked, "What's going on?" Shortly later, after an ultrasound, they found something on the right side and sent me to a cancer doctor. What they found was large enough to start testing right away.

My mother said, "When they tell you surgery, you tell them that you are going to insist on a complete hysterectomy." She didn't have a complete hysterectomy when she had hers, and she said that if she knew then what she knows now, she would have insisted that they take it all. When I was finally diagnosed, I was told I'd have to go to the cancer centre, because they don't have the technology in my city, and, yes, that I would have to have a complete hysterectomy.

I was angry, like anyone would be, at my family doctor. In fact, when he asked, I told my brother that my family doctor is about one-third of my size, so I could go into her office, knock her down, and sit on her. That got him to laugh. We weren't very pleased with this doctor anyway because she makes mistakes on prescriptions. Once she gave me the wrong strength for my leg medicine and it took her two months to get it right. She's also left patients without another attending doctor while she's been on holidays. And it's been hard to get files very quickly from her office.

"You'll Be Fine"

Since then, after the initial upset when I got the news that it was cancer, I haven't had many problems with it at all. When he did the biopsy, the doctor said, "It is my job to say the 'C word,' which is 'cancer'—ovarian cancer." He told me that it usually strikes women after the age of 50 years or after menopause, and I said to him, "Stuff happens and you have to deal with it."

He turned to me and said, "Good answer. You'll be fine."

When I got home, I had received an email note from my brother who lives in the States. He responded after he got Mom's note, and he asked me what does this mean, and what does this do? I said, "This is just something that we are going to have to deal with because stuff happens, and I can email you more information as we I get it."

He's one of four brothers I have. Three of them have nine children between them, so that cured me of ever wanting to have children. I have nine nieces and nephews.

I actually haven't had the surgery yet. My ovaries were both over six inches long, so they had to be reduced by chemotherapy. The larger they are, the harder they are to remove. One of the first things that they did at the cancer centre was drain some of the fluid off my stomach, which had never been done.

That does help my breathing. When I sleep at night I actually often snore, even if I sleep on my side, because of the pressure on my diaphragm. I can still get winded easily. It's not that bad at the moment, but I can get winded going up and down the stairs. But it can get pretty serious.

Soon I'll have my eighth treatment scan. I just finished the last chemo today, and soon the doctors and I will discuss surgery. Apparently I have now qualified for the surgery, but they haven't booked a date for it.

It's interesting, I have a friend who had a mother who had a cancer scare, and she has to go in every couple of years to have a CT scan or an ultrasound to make sure that everything is fine. Last year, a cyst formed on her ovary that burst and dispersed throughout her body. And everything is fine. Her doctor got in touch with her and said she now is a yearly patient—she has to get checked yearly. So I wondered, why didn't I ever have to have anything like that?

But my family and friends have been very supportive. All my relatives phone and use email. I have heard from some relatives that I have never even met before. I told everybody that I would keep them updated, and if nothing else I can describe my bald head. We come from the States originally. Between my aunt and my mom, a little message was sent to everyone about it, and people started responding. I got emails from everyone and anybody.

A best friend of hers from high school (who is also my dad's cousin), who had breast cancer said that if I need information about anything, support, or someone to talk to, she would be there for me. When I did get home, I emailed everybody and noted I will be going on a government drug plan, which means that I won't have to pay for this drug treatment that I am currently on. I have ovarian cancer and I will have to have chemo and surgery and more chemo, and they told me that if they told me all the information that they know, then my brain would melt and run out of my ears. So they give you a certain amount of information at a time.

On that first Monday of chemo, my dad, who used to work near the cancer centre, dropped me off on the way to work. My dad has since retired so he still drives me, and sometimes we visit my brother.

Side Effects ... and Green Hair

As of now, I have a blood clot in my leg. They now know enough about cancer treatments to know that all cancers are going to give you blood clots in your legs. And they are going to send you for a test for it every couple of weeks until they find it. I also now know that I shouldn't take the water pill that I was on, because it reacts to the chemo and causes a drug reaction. I was on a very minimal dosage of it anyway, and I didn't bring it with me, so it's not a problem.

I have lost my hair. It went down to peach fuzz after I started the standard treatments, and I was always wearing hats. I had six treatments, and then CT scans showed it wasn't working. I thought this was the case, because my hair started growing back. So I went on another treatment. I get no nausea. I get a little redness across my face that comes and goes.

Even today my nieces and nephews, the youngest who were just three years old when I first lost my hair, come and look at my hair. They are in the process of being adopted by my oldest brother. After my first treatment, the Monday after Mother's Day in 2002, we got together at my brother's place. My brother and his wife are actors, and she was going through some stuff from their acting stuff to give the kids something to play with. She found some eyebrow pencils and curlers from when her friend had chemo, and she gave them to me in case I ever needed them.

So when we got together I said, "Sure, curl my hair." It would be something fun to do.

And I went over to Mom after I got off of the phone, and she said, "Yes you have had curled hair before, but I was just thinking that you had never dyed it."

I said, "You know what? You're right. I never have."

They were going to the grocery, and I said, "Why don't you pick up some temporary hair colour of your choice, something easy to put on. We'll take that along and see what we can do."

So I went to chemo with green hair; as a matter of fact I have a picture of myself with green hair. It was from green hair dye. We put dollar store stuff in it, like daisies and butterflies. My sister-in-law also had some gel glitter that you could wipe on your clothes or your hair. So I went to chemo with emerald green hair with daisies and butterflies, and I was turning heads all over the place.

Mary's family celebrated her life 28 months after her diagnosis of ovarian cancer.

Bilgay

Keep your face to the sunshine
And you cannot see the shadow.
—Helen Keller

Bilgay loved her long-time work of helping care for newborns in a hospital nursery. But her life started changing when she felt unusual symptoms that doctors couldn't fully understand. Then her life turned upside down the night she found herself on the bathroom floor at her home. Her ovarian cancer was making its mark. Before long, this once socially active dynamo became a self-described "homey wife," with her good days and her bad days. "Sometimes I feel like I'm 80 years old," she said. "I have to just sit and be a blob for a little bit."

I WAS ILL FOR FOUR MONTHS before I was diagnosed. I think maybe that something should have been picked up at that time. I worked at the hospital in the nursery and I was off of work with a really high temperature, like 39 to 40 degrees, and I knew that it wasn't right. I had a rash all over my body, pinpoint red, from the neck down. The rash was very itchy, and I remember I went into work the next day and went into the emergency just to get checked out.

I didn't want to affect the babies that I was with—I was thinking of them. They said, "Oh, it's probably a viral thing," and I was thinking in my head, "That's not right, I am the healthiest person." They didn't even want to do a blood culture. Two days later, the rash had turned into what looked like bruises.

My doctor didn't know what to make of it, so he sent me to a specialist, and they checked everything out and thought that I had parvovirus. They were saying, "Isn't that what dogs get?" But it was something babies got, and it made sense that I contracted it from being around babies. But when they took the blood samples from me they found out that I did not have it. So they didn't do anything. Time went by and I got better. The rash cleared up.

But then my limbs got stiff—my arms, legs, and feet. I was like a stick person walking around. I couldn't get out of the tub, and I was splashing around like a whale. It went on for four months, and then it cleared up and I went to work again for a couple of days. Then on the weekend, I remember that I couldn't button up my pants. So no one picked up on it. Even the doctor I went to about my arms checked my stomach, and he said nothing about it. That's what blows me away.

I WENT TO THE FAMILY DOCTOR, and he said, "You have to go and have an ultrasound done." That same day he said to me, "It's not good news." Then your whole world falls apart.

At the cancer clinic, they are a compassionate group of people; I think that it is a prerequisite to working there. You are in the midst of this devastating disease, and they just take you into their arms. I think people in this situation need this. They would do anything for you.

The setback for me was that they discovered this at a time when I was super busy at the hospital, so they were telling me that I had to wait, and that I was on a waiting list. That was bad news, because when you know that this thing is in you, you just want to get it out. It was making me visibly sick. Anyway, we went home, and it wasn't until the following weekend that I really started to feel sick. I couldn't eat, and I think everything was backing up. And I am not a complainer. I don't just run to the hospital for anything. That's just my makeup. Maybe it's not a good way to be. I remember that night, everyone had gone to bed, and I felt that something wasn't going to go right. I had a premonition. I remember going to the bathroom, and I felt like everything was up to here, pushed up to my neck.

That evening, I remember calling the hospital, and they said, "Well, if you throw up come in," but I was feeling bad already. Maybe they said that because I sounded calm and I wasn't yelling or anything. Anyway, I remember I went to the bathroom and I sat on the toilet. I remember calling for my husband. I said, "I need you," and that was it. I passed out.

When I woke up, my husband was on top of me doing cardiac massage. I guess with the panic he didn't know what to do. I remember waking up and saying, "What are you doing? Take your hands off of me!"

I was still disoriented, and all I kept thinking about was the kids. I remember thinking, "Here I am lying on the floor without my pants—the kids are going to come running in and see me without my underwear," and I am thinking, "I have to get my pants on." So, I'm pulling my pants up, and then I threw up. Then I was worried about the rug. I didn't want to shock the family—I was doing everything to make it normal, so they wouldn't see. I was protecting them.

Then they called the ambulance and that's how I got in. I have a true belief that someone higher up was watching me. I still believe that if I hadn't passed out, I would still be on the waiting list. So it was a good thing that I passed out. It got my cleansing surgery. I was in intensive care for a few days because I lost a lot of blood. I remember they stuck a tube up my nose that went to my stomach, and I was in there for several days.

My oldest daughter stayed there with me. She is 19 years old now. She stayed every night with me so I wouldn't be by myself. But you know, what a hectic thing—when a mother is removed from a household, it just falls apart. And you are so worried about what is going on at home. Everyone says that I look wonderful, but they don't know what goes on in here, and in my heart. The heartache is still there.

So I got through that, and then I remember being on the ward—my doctor was away, and the other doctor who was covering for him was such a gentle man, he reminded me of my brother. He wanted to take the tube out, and I said, "Don't rush, just give it another few days."

He made such a strange face and wondered why I didn't want to take it out, and then one day he came in and said, "That's it. Today's the day that we are taking out the tube." Then I said, "Okay, today's the day."

I have had wonderful care—I just can't say enough. I came home after the surgery, and I had my first chemo and I became occluded again, and then I had to go back in. They have to cleanse you, to get your bowels working again. I remember I was in a ward, and the poor lady who was in the room with me, I felt so sorry for her—I think that she had lost her mind. But I can understand it better now. She wanted to go home; I don't know why she couldn't. One day, about 13 of them were holding her on her stretcher; it was very upsetting to me. I went to the sunroom to get out of the room, and I slept in the sunroom. It was very upsetting to me, but I understand that they had to do what they did for her health.

You have to have such faith in them and the system. My VON nurses [Victorian Order of Nurses] have been wonderful, and I have been involved with a social worker from the very beginning. She is my strength—she understands me now, and she can tell me how I feel before I tell her. I feel very fortunate to have her.

I find that sometimes for the family, the cancer is all a bit overwhelming. I remember when I was first diagnosed, I used to cry all the time. When they told me I was disease free, I cried for a year. I couldn't even do anything. I thought that I could go back to work—that was my dream—and I couldn't even do that. So they gave me time, and that was so good; they didn't force me to do anything that I wasn't ready to do. It was just my mind. When I was on the treatments I was okay. I had something to concentrate on.

But once they took that away, I had nothing left, and I felt lost. I put my family through terrible things; I cried and cried. My husband thought that I was losing it. I expected so much from him, but he was afraid of me. You are afraid of getting close, so you take two steps back. But I didn't want him to be backing off—I wanted him to move forward. I have had to wait more than two years for him to stop stepping back. That's a long wait. He has a motorcycle, and he would vent through that. He would leave in the evening, and we would never have our family dinners together anymore. I would say, "What is this?"

We were so family-oriented, but we wouldn't do that anymore. He would leave, and I would ask, "Where are you going?" He would leave for hours on end, and he would phone me from another city, just to tell me that he loved me. He wouldn't tell me to my face—he would tell me from a distance. It took me a long time. My social worker helped me to understand what was going on in his head.

I am sure that he still is afraid, but at least now he is spending more time at home. He is not taking off like he used to. That was so upsetting to me; I used to cry, and no one knows what to say. His mother would come down, and what was she going to say to him? He's her son, and the circle goes round and round. The kids were upset, and they would say to him, "What did you say to her?" And it goes around and around. It was terrible.

Then one day I thought I'd better get myself together, because this is not good, what I am doing. I took responsibility. It took a little while, and I still cry on some days. But you know now, I tell my social worker, they don't see me as much—I do it in my own spare time. I am trying to make it as normal as possible.

My daughter is 20 this year, and my other daughter will be 18, and then I have a 12-year-old, and my little guy, my surprise in life, will be 7 years old in two weeks.

My family is number one to me. Just like getting up in the morning, I have a routine; I get up for them to go to school in the morning, no matter how tired I am. I have my hair done. I stick to my routine—I do it every single day.

I am Catholic, and I have a girl who pops in. I used to work with this girl years ago, and all of a sudden she just pops in. She starts talking to me about the Bible. I don't know the Bible that well, but she helps me to understand what it says. I believe in the Bible and in the Catholic religion. But here's a girl that just popped into my life. That's what I am saying: there are so many people that have come into my life. We have to be open to letting these people into our lives. I think sometimes when we are so injured and so hurt, we want to go away and hide.

I don't go to group meetings. Occasionally, if I am at the clinic I meet someone, or if I go to my CT scans I meet people who are there for a similar things, and I start chatting to them. I think they enjoy talking to me, because I feel more comfortable talking about it now. It has taken me a long time to get here. I am okay with it. I feel them out first, and then if they ask me something, we go ahead from there.

When I was diagnosed I was at stage three, and I couldn't understand how I could get to that stage so quickly because I have never been sick before in my life. And it is now in my lymph nodes and in my stomach area. I understand it as a nurse, but as a patient I find it upsetting. I have two ways of thinking: both nurse and patient. I am still staying hopeful because you have to; if you don't, everything will fall apart. And I have good days and bad days. I am in chemo now, so I am really tired. My concentration is gone because of the stress and the chemo. I tell the kids that they have to tell me things a couple of times before it will sink in. I still can't sleep at night; I take things to help me relax. I take pills to make me regular, and I haven't had any more problems for more than two years. My doctor says if it works for me, I should go ahead and take it, and that's the way I feel. I don't overdo it every day—it's only when I have a problem.

It wasn't until a couple of months ago, when they gave me a pain pill to take, that I figured out that I even had pain, because it isn't like a pounding headache—it is more like a deep, gnawing pain. I just didn't feel good, and I just didn't know what it was, until the doctor said to try this and I felt better.

I would tell people how important it is to get to a doctor as quick as they can. I say to people that you don't know how many people are in the same boat until you walk through those doors. People who have no one that is ill have no idea. Heavens, when you walk through that door every clinic is full. What an eye opener. It is like that every day, and that is just one centre. How many other centres are like that?

I do miss work. I loved what I did. I used to tell people that those were my babies, and when I worked there for 12 hours those *were* mine. Yes, I miss them. But I have been very lucky that I have been given time to be with my family because my husband and I used to work opposite shifts all the time. It was great for the kids, but we never got to see each other. It was like that for 25 years. So in a way I am blessed now because I get to be a homey wife. No, I am enjoying it. So this is my time in life to do this. And it is busy enough with what is going on. I don't think that my mind is there anymore to go back to work, so this is just right for me now.

I think the chemicals change you. They go everywhere. I remember when I had my first bout of treatments and I was off for a year, and then it came back and I had my second bout of treatments, I developed an allergy to one of the chemo drugs. I wanted to scratch my skin off. When I went to the bathroom and put water on my skin, it got worse and worse, and I thought that I had to say something now because it wasn't going away. Then when I told them, they all went into a panic. And you know why I was afraid to say anything? I was afraid that they would stop the medication. I thought that I would rather take a chance and say nothing but get that medication in me. I was going to fight to the end.

I often wonder what I would have done without my worker. Who would I have to talk to? The VON nurses just come and do their job and then they leave, but she stays and talks. She said that her hours have been cut back, and I think that this is a very important service that people really need. The mental and emotional needs are important; it keeps you from going insane. If you just thought about the eventual outcome, you would go insane. I can't even imagine the people who don't have anyone to talk to. I remember when my husband and I were having such a hard time and I had to learn to back off. He was just so overwhelmed by it, he would say, "What is this? Everything is you, you, you!"

And I didn't see it that way. Well, of course it's me. I was just trying to pull him back to me, and I didn't know how to do that. Everyone's got his or her coping mechanisms. My kids have never run from me. And on my side, I have four brothers. One emails me all the time and says, "What's happening?" The one here phones me. And on my husband's side, he has a younger brother who phones me all the time. The others keep their distance, and you can understand that. They are afraid; they don't know what to say.

I am the only girl in my family. My mother died of breast cancer, but she left it too long. She was only 40 years old when she died. I was around 16 years old, and I just remember that heartache. I want to spare my children that heartache. That is why I am feeling that I need to keep everyone together for as long as I can. I don't want them to feel what I felt. I also lost my dad a year later from a heart attack. So you learn to cope. My brothers and I just stuck it out.

Losing my hair was so devastating. You don't know how much your crowning glory means to you. It was after my Taxol, my second treatment. I remember I went into the shower and I went to wash it very lightly and a whole bunch came out, so I wrapped my head up. I wouldn't let anyone see me like that. Isn't that silly? So I had my wig, and I went around with that. It grows back very well. I remember going to that Look Good Feel Better program, and I thought that it was a great thing. My two older children came with me and we were all in it together. They made it fun with samples, and it was so special.

I do my thing in the morning, and then I lie down, do the laundry, lie down, make dinner, and then lie down again. It is harder now that I am in chemo because all my energy is drained. Usually you feel better the second week. I remember when I was on my first round of chemo and my little guy went to school on alternate days, I thought I was a supermom and could do anything. So I took him to the park, two blocks down, and I couldn't move. I just lay on the bench while he played in the sand. You think you can do all this, but you can't; you feel all right, and then it hits you and you have to lie down. Even when you think you are okay, you aren't okay. I just do enough and then I rest. It is important to rest. A lot of people don't think about it—they don't know how important it is to rest. Now I have to. Sometimes I feel like I am 80 years old. I have to just sit and be a blob for a little bit.

Bilgay journeyed 56 months with ovarian cancer.

Denise

As long as there is someone who loves us,
We will remain alive.
Memories make us immortal.
In truth, love will outlive even memories.

—Leo F. Buscaglia

Denise was always a woman of energy. A former high school teacher who then taught preschool for 20 years, she loved her job. But after she found out she had ovarian cancer, her new life spelled retirement. Now, a church Sunday-school class is among the networks that keep her going—plus her husband and two daughters. They help encourage her to take a mindset of staying as active as possible. She puts it plainly: "You can't give up; you have to keep fighting, and try to keep going."

MY STORY STARTED IN THE LATE summer, early fall, when I had what I thought were a lot of bladder infections, but the tests kept coming back that it wasn't that. So they did an ultrasound and sent me to a urologist. He said that everything looked fine, that I had fibroids, but people live with those for years. He said that I had freckles on my kidneys, "but don't let anybody tell you those are a problem." But after Christmas I started losing weight, and I wasn't feeling 100 percent. Then by February and the beginning of March, I was getting some bloating around my middle and I thought: middle-age spread.

I was busy, I was working and doing all my volunteer work, and I just kept going. Then by mid-March it was sore, and I thought, something is wrong, and that's when I went to the doctor. They said that there was a cyst. He said, "Don't worry about it—we will just do a hysterectomy," and he booked that for the end of March. And after the operation, he said, "I don't like what I saw, but don't worry I have been wrong before—we will get the results back." Well, then, a couple of weeks later, he called me back and said that it was cancer and that he couldn't answer any questions but the cancer clinic would be contacted.

And that's how I found out. Out of the blue, I picked up the phone and they said, "Hello, this is Dr. so and so, and I have some bad news for you." And then I had to wait until I got to the clinic to find out what was going on.

They referred me to the cancer clinic, and it was a gynecologic oncologist I saw there. The treatment started very quickly. She explained to me about the clinical trial, and I agreed to do that. So we went from there. We did the clinical trial and that was about eight months. It didn't work, so then we were trying another drug before Christmas. She said that it wasn't working, that the cancer is going to kill you. So we came home and cried all weekend.

Then we said, "Look, that's not who we are, and what we are. We are not going to give up. We will do what we can; we will try the new drug."

I have two things going for me, I think, in this whole process: first of all I tend to be a positive person, and secondly I have very strong faith. These two things have stood me in very good stead through all of this.

I am Presbyterian. I was raised Anglican, and when I got married 30 some-odd years ago, I changed to Presbyterian. I found that I have wonderful friends and a wonderful support system. The first drug that I was on, I had to go five days a week every three weeks. I had to get rides up there, and I never had a problem. The phone would start ringing and someone would offer to take me all the time. People have offered rides, made food, and helped when I have been really down. Quite often it's a Monday when I am all by myself, and those are the days when my neighbour drops in or my aunt drops in, and then I just carry on. The last month has been hard because I was in the hospital with blood clots in my leg and it went to my lungs, plus I had stomach problems and I had thrush and I had too much calcium in my blood, so I don't have much energy. That really bothers me because I am normally a high-energy person.

I have two daughters, and they are also both high-energy people. My oldest daughter lives about an hour away, and our youngest daughter lives here. It is nice to have them close. The girls are good about keeping in touch with me.

Our oldest daughter is getting married this summer. She is converting to Judaism—her husband is Jewish. She has been at it since last year. We certainly like her husband, so we support her decision. She is a very determined, strong-willed young lady, so we have no reservations that anyone is pushing her into it.

MY FRIENDS LAUGH AT ME because they say that before I had super energy, and now I just have normal energy. I spend quite a bit of time lying on the couch now. I am working through that. I don't know whether it's the clots and the healing of the lungs that are causing this. I'm doing blood thinners; I was on Coumadin for a while. My own doctor said that it was the lungs that are still healing. I must admit, the wind and the cold weather just about do me in right now.

They did the hysterectomy, and I'm now on this particular chemotherapy drug. This is number four. My doctor is going to evaluate and see. My understanding initially was that I could have up to eight of these. She has also put me on a list for another clinical trial. We just take one step at a time. I just go once a month right now, and so I go in next week.

Initially my family reacted the same way that I did and said, "Let's do something about this and get rid of it." My husband knows the whole story. My kids know that the drugs were not working. That's all we have told them, and that we are trying some more drugs. Because my oldest daughter is getting married in the summer, we are trying to make that the focus of our lives right now. She hasn't coped that well. She has struggled with this. There is a lot of history with her, and that is why it's upsetting her even more.

My husband works at the steel factory. He's a planner and has worked for 33 years. He's coping, and he is very good at helping. It has been very hard on everyone in the family, particularly my husband because he knows that this may not have a good ending. And now he just had a colonoscopy and they removed a polyp. He just went to get the results, and the doctor said, "You are one lucky man."

Apparently there was some cancer on the polyp, but it hadn't got to the soft tissue yet, so he said as far as he can tell, my husband is cured. So we got some good news. My husband's dad died last February of colorectal cancer; his uncle died, his grandmother died, all of colorectal cancer. My family is not the one with cancer—it's all his. I think that this has hit him a little harder because of all that has happened in the past year. But in my family there is no cancer, just heart disease or stroke. So I'm after my girls to keep on top of it. This is why it was quite the shock for us.

MY HERITAGE IS GERMAN AND BRITISH, and my husband's is Irish and Ukrainian. We have been here for a few generations.

I taught a preschool program for 20 years, and before that I taught high school. Both my girls are teachers too. I loved my job and I took a leave of absence, but this fall I had to resign or retire. I miss it, but I still have my Sunday-school class, and that keeps me going because I miss them. I'm happy to have such a good network of support.

For someone who was just diagnosed, I'd say, "You can't give up—you have to keep fighting and try to keep going." I guess it would have helped to talk to people with ovarian cancer about what they are going through. I don't think that I was ready for it initially—I just wanted to get on with it and tackle it. The more I get into it, I think it is more valuable.

Up until January I was doing it all. At Christmas I did it all. I shopped, I wrapped, I baked, I cleaned, I cooked, I entertained, I visited relatives. We had a very nice, busy Christmas, and I loved it. Up until that point there were some days that I was tired and had to have a nap. Since this bout in early January and since I came home from the hospital I haven't done a lot. I have to figure out what is going on because I hate this. I tried to get out at least once a day, but yesterday and today I couldn't have cared less.

Usually I go with people. I did venture out on Monday by myself to get the girls their Valentine presents. My husband was going to be working late and my daughter was coming Monday night, and I knew what I wanted to get. It was the first time I had driven in a month, and I just drove down to the store, picked up their gifts, and drove back. It made me feel good that I could do that. It's the walking that is tiring, not the driving.

Next Friday, I will have the chemo and I have to get more fragments. Then I have a CT scan to evaluate where we are. I have been very impressed with the speed in which things have happened, and I certainly like my doctor. I have been pleased that way. I worked with the clinical trials nurse for a while and I thought the world of her—she is just a sweetheart. I miss her now. She was working with the clinical trial for the first eight months. She was so caring, and you could ask her anything and she would tell you. That is the secret when you are first diagnosed: to have someone to talk to. The doctors often don't have time, and they are in and out. Sometimes there is a nurse, but I see a different one all the time. So you don't build up the same rapport. The support made a difference initially when I first started the treatment.

I never felt a lot of pain or anything. I did get out of breath, and that's what triggered me that there was something wrong. I am not sure whether it is because of the lungs that I get tired, or if it is a bit of a mental thing too, where this is the time of year when I don't have to do anything. Once I got out I did enjoy it, but it is hard to get myself moving to go out.

I haven't travelled since I've been ill. We used to travel to the Caribbean and to Mexico. I said to my husband before Christmas I would dearly love to get away, even just overnight, but he didn't seem to think that is urgent right now. He said that the spring would be better. I just need something to look forward to, a change of scenery. Not just the blood work.

Denise enjoyed her Caribbean cruises during 15 months with ovarian cancer.

Sarah

... sore must be the storm
That could abash the little Bird
That kept so many warm

—from "'Hope' Is the Thing with Feathers,"
   by Emily Dickinson

Sarah had a long history of illnesses, some of which led to infertility. But when ovarian cancer hit in her early 40s and then recurred, everything changed for her, her two adopted girls, and her other loved ones. Sarah admits she's a compulsive worrier. Yet she found a unique spirit of optimism when she needed it. In addition to her family, a new friendship and therapeutic journaling were supports that carried her. And in the end, she was reminded that she needed to give everything to her Maker, by simply living one day at a time.

I'M 42 YEARS OLD, BORN AND raised in moderate-sized city. My parents are both in this area, and they have been a wonderful support. I have one brother, who is younger than I am. There has been a bit of bowel and colon cancer in our family, but no ovarian cancer. My oldest daughter is 8 years old, and my other daughter is 6.

I'm also an office manager. Because of fatigue, I have cut back my hours. Luckily, I have a boss who is willing to work with me, and I also do some job-sharing with another lady who is flexible picking up hours when I can't make it in.

I've always had health problems. Even when I was a teenager I suffered from menstrual pain and discomfort. Then in my early 20s I was diagnosed with endometriosis. Through ages 18 to 25, I had a couple of scopes down and they burned off some of the scar tissue. I had reconstructive surgery because we were trying to have children, but it wasn't working out. They did surgery because my fallopian tubes were mushed together with the endometriosis and the scar tissue and whatnot. So that was done hoping to open up the tubes. Unfortunately, it didn't work and infertility resulted. So we adopted the kids, and after that I had a hysterectomy, in 2000.

When I started having the pain I was doing a lot of walking, but I couldn't figure out what was going on. So I went to the doctor and they discovered that there was indeed a mass. They ordered a CT scan the next day, and within a week I had surgery. The doctors didn't really know what they were dealing with because I had a total hysterectomy. They didn't know what they were going in to look at. But they discovered a mass. They took it out, found that it was cancer, and set up follow-up treatments for me at the cancer centre.

Welcoming Arms

I feel totally that I'm in welcoming arms in the health care system over there. The nurses and doctors are superb. I had a couple rounds of chemotherapy, and then they decided to go in and do surgery again. They went into my stomach and wanted to make sure that yes, indeed, they did get it all, because there was an ovarian cell that must have been left behind or went undetected with the first surgery. So that went bad, because that ovarian cell left behind turned into the ovarian cancer.

So they did the surgery and said everything was fine. I finished my six rounds of chemo. Everything was done on the side of precaution. They wanted to make sure they got it all because when they were removing the mass it broke. So it broke in my abdomen. That was another reason that they wanted to go back in and make sure.

I was cancer free for about six months, but I started having a little more pain. So I went back, and sure enough there was a return of the cancer. Now I am undergoing chemo treatments once again. They found that they weren't getting anywhere, the cancer was spreading, and so what they have done—they are very proactive—is put me on this study. I am feeling 100 percent better. The doctors have been so positive from the get-go. When I was told that it was back, I automatically thought of dying. The fear came back. But this time it was like we had many options. The doctors were not saying this is it. They were so positive in reinforcing this in my head. It has made a huge impact on my outlook.

The study means that I go to the cancer centre one day a week for three weeks and get an infusion of protein. It's 90 minutes the first time, then one hour. Yesterday I was cut back to 30 minutes. Now I go down every other week. In addition to the infusion, I am taking my chemotherapy tablet every day.

In the past two weeks I have felt the best that I have felt in a long time. There is still some fatigue there, but as far as side effects, no. I am feeling awesome. You have to go and lie down when you are tired and learn your limitations, which I am doing now. It's been good. I don't feel like I've been taken over by the process at all. If I were to say that I don't want to do this anymore, that would be fine.

The doctors keep me informed and are more than willing to answer questions. They are wonderful. It's awesome—even in the chemo lab yesterday they were so understaffed and running like crazy, yet they still take that time to talk to you as a person. And there have been many times that I have been there and crying, and they are there 100 percent. So you really don't feel like a number.

Raw Emotions and the Hope Factor

I did attend a support group meeting at the hospice, but it was just after I had got my clean bill of health, so I found that the timing wasn't right. It was like I had attained victory. I had fought it, and now it was like, "Wow! Time to carry on with life!" It changes you. So when I went, the support group brought me down because I could relate to what everyone was saying. My emotions were so raw still, it was just too much. I am just a little bit past that, and I have got to go and find some hope and find the light again. I couldn't attend any of those. There is another support group, and I am debating whether I want to do that again. I am not sure.

It's so cliché, when people say that it is a life-altering situation. It really is, but I think until you really experience it and have it under your belt, it's hard to get the full concept of it all. The first big shock was when the doctors came in and said that they got the pathology back and that it was cancer. Another one was when I went to the cancer centre and they told me that I had to have surgery again and I had to have chemo. All of those were huge. Those moments just seem to freeze.

Going through this, my coping skills are much better than they used to be. You are given so much to handle, and it's like, "Oh my gosh." Then you have those thoughts of death, and talk about getting overwhelmed!

I have learned that "one day at a time" is so helpful in getting through it. Before, I wouldn't look at one day at a time. I would look at one week at a time or a month at a time. Now it is a totally different way of looking at life. It's one day at a time. There are so many hours in a day, and now I think that there is so much living you can do in one day if you just look at it as one day at a time.

For me, that's key. If I can stay with that philosophy then I find that my coping skills are better and it keeps everything in perspective. Just the little things; like people say, don't sweat the small stuff. That kind of stuff is so true. Just valuing conversations with people is important. It just brings everything into a new perspective.

Then there's the hope factor. Through this whole thing I have gone through so many different emotions, so many phases of hope. From no hope and despair, and then finally you make it and you think you have got it. Then it comes back again and you kind of get through that. And now I think I am learning how to live with it on a daily basis and appreciating the blessings that I do have, not the things that I don't have. I don't think I will ever be the same physically or emotionally after all this.

You are changed because you have gone through so much. I think it is a great emotional growth or spiritual growth that happens inside, that you can't help but look at life differently. And people. When you walk into that hospital, that cancer clinic, as much as I hate going there, I always come out feeling so blessed because there is always somebody worse off. I walk out of there thinking, you know, I have got the day. I am still here, still breathing. It could be a whole lot worse. So you just have to find the good and the blessings, and some days it is hard.

Of course, I've been too hard on myself too. I think that it is such a learning experience because you learn so much about yourself, your limitations, and who is important in your life—your family, your friends, and the support that is there. It just really brings the whole thing into focus, what I want my world to be about. If I were to go tomorrow, I know who and what I would surround myself with. And it has been the people that have been here for me through thick and thin, and those people down at the cancer centre. It just brings a whole new appreciation and a whole new outlook. It's uplifting and it's an awesome feeling.

A New Sister

For me, my faith has played a role too. The support that I have received through the church, from friends, and my ability to stay focused have helped to strengthen my ability to go one day at a time. I was raised Catholic. I went to church all the time but didn't really know what it was about. I was confirmed but really didn't understand it. Then about one and a half years before this all started, I met a friend. She planted the seed and got me interested in church. I always thought that there was something different about this lady, and I just wanted more of that, and it was all good. So then we connected, and lo and behold, she has an important role in all this.

Now we are like sisters. We truly believe that we were God-given to each other, because our relationship is awesome. She drew me to the church, faith, and all that. And she has connected me with all the people who have helped me in so many ways. On those days when I can't get off the couch, just emotionally, it has been my faith and her reassurance in that faith that have helped me through.

Now I kind of have to wonder where I would be without it, because it is so important to me. This girlfriend is like my spiritual mentor. It's just an awesome story. Actually, I'm in the midst of writing a bit of a book. It starts with her and me and our relationship, and how we were brought together. It's going to be spiritually based. I was journaling this whole experience.

The journaling has been awesome, really therapeutic. I wrote and wrote the whole time, so I have notes and notes and feelings on paper. Then I thought, I want to compile this because my children have been such a key part of this and I want them to know when they get older how important they were. I have had to hold up on the writing, and again I think it is timing; it just doesn't feel right at this time, but when it feels right I am going to get back at it.

My daughters are very intuitive little creatures. We found from the very start it was best to be honest with them, because they are very curious and they will ask. So we told them that Mommy had a sore in her stomach and that hopefully the doctors would help. I always bring God into it, so God is there. They were good. They were upset, to say the least. And so was I. And in the beginning I really was torn about whether to show them my emotions or not. Do I hold back?

We worked our way through that, and I showed emotions and they would just come running whenever they could tell, sometimes even before, I was going to cry. Our littlest one would bring the Kleenex box and say, "Here, Mom," and give me hugs. I found the roles were reversed and they were the mom and I was the little kid. They were patting me on the back, saying, "Mom, you are going to be okay," and that sort of thing.

On the days when I was on the couch they would bring me art with "We love you, Mom." I have it framed downstairs. They were the hope and strength for me. I would just wait for them. I mean, days were spent here looking out the window until they would come in after school yelling, "Mom, Mom, Mom!" That's what it's all about.

So yes, they have been really good, really supportive. And they are resilient. When I had to go back to chemo a second time, it wasn't as tough on them. We said, again, "Mommy's got to have some down days again." And they were okay with it. They were like, "Okay, Mom, we'll be there again."

This time around, it was almost a breeze to them. I just found that it brings out their emotions, and they just show so many more emotions now than they did before. If somebody says something, they say, "Oh, Mommy is just not feeling good today" or whatever, and they understand that. They know I can't always get up and do something or play. Sometimes they get frustrated, but on the whole they are really good with that. I think is it best, you know, just being upfront and honest with them. They have played a huge role.

Sometimes you lose that desire to carry on and to keep going. But my two girls have given me a reason to want to carry on through those dark days. My husband has been so positive too. He has a great sense of humour, and those are two things that you really appreciate.

There are days. I have had them and there is just no getting around them. I couldn't quite figure out how you do it, but you just keep putting one foot in front of the other. My girlfriend keeps saying baby steps will get you through it. It was only about a month ago that I realized I am getting through it; I didn't think that I ever could. My journals, when I re-read them, tell me that I have been through a lot, the emotional side of it all. And they tell me that I am still here.

One Day at a Time

All through this I kept saying, "I can't do this, I can't do this." And everybody kept saying, "Yes, you can. Yes, you can."

All this has strengthened me as an individual. I think it's that desire to be still in control that leads you to that little struggle back and forth.

On those days where I can give it to God and I can say, "It's yours," then my days are so much better. So when you can do it, it's awesome. But I give and take. That's only me. I mean, he wants it all.

I wear this medallion around my neck that says "one day at a time." And on the back is the Serenity Prayer. And, what if I had all the wisdom just to give it over all the time? But I think that it is human nature to want to have a sense of control. Still, it's this fear of death that has strengthened my faith. And when I have those overwhelming fears of losing my family, that's when my faith really has to strengthen in order to cope with it. So yes, my faith is huge. We aren't in control, and I am living proof that we aren't.

Before this I was a real worrier—I worried about everything—so when I was cancer free I found that I was worrying a lot about what if it comes back? I had six months when it wasn't there, and through those six months I was struggling with what-ifs. And now that it has come back, I have realized that you can't prepare yourself for it. So you might as well take the worry out of it and give it over. It makes the time that you do have so much more enjoyable. It sounds so cliché, but it is so true.

When I was diagnosed originally, people kept saying, "Why are you not angry? What's with this?" And you know what? Had I not been walking as much as I had walked that time when I was having the pain, it wouldn't have been brought to my attention. And had I not had a body that talks to me, the doctors have said that I could have been coming in five years from now and we could be saying that it is too late.

I was also having pain because of a bowel problem, and if I didn't have that, the ovarian cancer could have taken over and I might not be here today. So it was sort of through another thing that they found the mass. I look at it as a blessing in disguise.

Do I blame anybody? No, there isn't any point in blaming anyone. It's just wasted energy. That is negative and you have to focus on the positive. I just look at it and say, "This is all faith related now for me." It just opened my world up to faith, to God, to the people at the church, and to an outside world that I had never really known about in such a huge way. This whole thing has been faith related, and my book will be based on God's love and how it has all played a role.

My change of direction in life has been all for the good. It's broadened new relationships with even my own parents. My dad and I are now closer than we have ever been. The relationship with my brother is also changed. Not only do these family members see me going through it, they are going through it too. It changes not only me, but the people who are around me. I see it as all for the good.

You know, when I am having days that are horrible, I tell my family. And they certainly know that. They are being positive as well. We are just enjoying the time that we have. And we keep saying to one another, "One day at a time." It just keeps going back to that. It's "You know what? Let's just focus on today."

Sarah walked for 29 months with ovarian cancer.

Patricia

All, everything that I understand
I understand only because I love

—from *War and Peace*, by Leo Tolstoy

Patricia hadn't been in hospital since she was a child with tonsillitis. But one mid-summer day when she was 49 years old, a mysterious pain hit her side. A pulled muscle perhaps? Four months later, she found out the truth: ovarian cancer. With three of her seven siblings having already died from unnatural causes, she faced the disease head on. And through the hell of it all, she found some unknown strength through faith in God, her husband, and friends from a newly discovered church.

I FIRST DISCOVERED SOMETHING wrong on a July 7 when I had a pain in my side. I waited a couple of weeks to see if it would go away, but it didn't. I went to my family doctor and he decided that it was probably a pulled muscle or something like that. So he sent me to a specialist who determined it was a pulled muscle, that I had pulled the muscle away from a rib. She gave me some painkillers and said that this would probably last about six weeks. I said, "Well, you know that it has already lasted about six weeks." She said, "Oh well, sometimes it lasts a little bit longer."

So it got worse. The painkillers were ineffective. So I went back to my family doctor, and a specialist then booked me for a CT scan and an ultrasound in case it was gallbladder related. It was another six weeks until the CT scan, and the pain was getting very intense. This was October by this time. Finally, in the first week in October, I said I just couldn't take it anymore, the pain was too intense. So with that my husband drove me into emergency and they started doing the tests. It was then around

Thanksgiving before they determined with blood tests and the CT scan that it was ovarian cancer. From there they shipped me off to the cancer centre, and there I started the chemotherapy.

With that they scheduled chemotherapy. It was carboplatin and Taxol. The combination of those two was supposed to run for six sessions. So we did three of these sessions and then there was surgery scheduled, and then we did the other three sessions. We got to five sessions, and the doctor determined that it was ineffective and that the tumour was still growing. In surgery, the doctors removed quite a large tumour but said that there were many more small tumours on the bowels.

The chemo didn't kill the cancer that had spread, so we waited another month and started the Taxol. That was ineffective as well. There is one more thing that we tried, a pill form that is usually used with breast cancer. The problem was that I couldn't keep anything down. The tumour is blocking my bowels, so I have a stomach-drain into a bag. I have to lock it off for an hour to absorb some of this pill. So we are just in the process of trying this pill, although this is the last resort. They can't do another surgery because it is too spread in my bowels, and the doctor says it would destroy my bowels.

I DON'T HAVE ANY CHILDREN. And while there are eight kids in my family, none of them have any cancer. My dad died of cancer, but it was Hodgkin's disease. They said that was unrelated to my cancer. They said mine was coming from the same genetic defect as breast cancer. Other than that, my aunt had died of breast cancer and I had another aunt who died of lung cancer, both sisters of my mom. As well, a brother, my uncle on my mom's side, died of throat cancer. But no ovarian cancer anywhere.

One of my siblings died of suicide. My eldest brother was a schizophrenic as well, and although they diagnosed it as suicide, I don't think that it was. I had another sister who was killed by a drunk driver, so I have lost three of my siblings.

But personally, I had never been in hospital other than for my tonsils when I was 12. I worked in payroll, benefits, and pension administration, and I was totally healthy all the time. But then I started feeling more tired, stressed, and overweight. And there was also lot of pain associated with my tumour. And there still is, because I am on permanent painkillers.

The oncologist said that I probably had the tumour for two years. I was kind of surprised by that as well. They took my uterus and my ovaries and a huge tumour, and that was supposed to solve most of the problem. The tumour they took out was the size of a football and was pushing up on one lung so I couldn't breathe. It actually caused the one lung not to work properly. It had fluid on it, and it led to me getting pneumonia while in hospital.

And now I can't even eat. I haven't eaten for a couple of months now. I just drink water. I have no nutrition. I take saline, that's all that I have. That has been several months.

The last few months have been very hard. Surgery was last December, and everything that possibly could go wrong did. I was supposed to be in the hospital two to three days tops, but was in for seventeen days. I finished chemo in the middle of February and kind of rode out March. In the middle of April, we went out West for my mother's 90th birthday. My husband and I got married while we were there. Near the end we almost didn't go because I was feeling so bad, just dragged down with pain. I was pretty sick the whole time that we were there. I ended up in the hospital throwing up, and they determined there was another tumour blocking my bowel.

I got back home and got nursing attention, but the tumour was back in less than two months. And based on that they determined that the previous chemo did nothing. So I have another tumour the size of a football on my bowel. I went through the second chemo with the second drug of choice, the Topotecan, which has done virtually nothing.

So for the past three months, since April, I have had nothing to eat. In the beginning I had something to eat, but 10 minutes later would throw up. Eventually I ended up in the hospital with complete renal failure, with kidneys shut down because of dehydration. I drink water like a fish and continually throw it all up. Since then, all I get is intravenous with saline to keep hydrated. And they're continuously draining my stomach because otherwise I throw up bile.

A Surprising Faith

Through all this, faith in God has been very helpful. Looking to God, I have something to lean on. This is very strange really because that wasn't always the case. But a friend of ours asked us to go to a program called Alpha. It's a 10-week course where you learn about God. You get answers to any questions that you may have had mulling around in the back of your head. It's a forum to answer these kinds of questions. So we went to learn more information. We were just learning this information for a couple of weeks when I was diagnosed.

As my husband points out, it turned into two journeys: one about discovering God, and the other about the overwhelming love and support that we have received from the wonderful people involved with church. My husband says this probably saved us, because without it, there would be just him and me.

My family is pretty much all out West. My husband's family is wonderful and they are all focused here. Although they try, they are not as involved as the people in the church. There were several people who had cancer, and I was even diagnosed at the same time as someone else in my Alpha group. So there was even a closer bond with the people in my church. And we need that, because a roller coaster of emotions comes with the territory. You try to be as hopeful as you can, but you have to feel both sides of the coin all the time.

Even in terms of sleep, I am up every couple of hours. And yet the oncologist is just as amazed. He says that he can't believe I have my muscle. "You look healthy and no one would believe that you are sick." And I am going, "Yeah, whatever."

When my husband rushed me to the hospital and explained to the doctor in emergency that I was being treated for ovarian cancer and a blocked bowel, he said that this was impossible because nobody could be that sick and look this good! Another doctor actually looked in my ear and suspected an inner ear infection because of my light-headedness and vomiting. That was the day that I was diagnosed with kidney failure.

And when they took me from the community hospital to the cancer centre hospital, they stuck me in intensive care and said that I had a 1 percent chance of getting out of there alive. So the doctors are limited, even by their own egos, if you will. You are often telling them what is going on and they are not listening. But they do have a tough job.

My husband says that after spending months at that cancer ward in the hospital, he used to feel kind of negative about the doctors and feel like they didn't know what they were doing. But after spending months in that cancer ward with women who are deathly ill, he can now appreciate how a doctor looks at a body, not the person. The one moment that doctor recognizes that there is a person there, he would not be able to do his job anymore.

People have encouraged me to keep a journal about my experiences, but I just haven't had the energy. That takes some actual prolonged enthusiasm, and it has just knocked me for a loop, so that I can barely just sleep. I sleep, I get up. I have 15 or 20 minutes sometimes when I have some energy, and then I go back to bed. Although I may look healthy, writing it down is not something I can advance to yet.

It's all been difficult. The chemo is a nasty bit of business. You suffer worse with that than you did from the cancer, in hopes of getting better. But unfortunately in our case it has been a downhill slide. It has been a struggle to try to live a life, go to somebody's birthday party, church on Sunday, or these Alpha meetings once a week; everything is a struggle. You give one hour and it takes a day to recover from that, and that's one of the sad parts of the whole thing.

After 12 months with ovarian cancer, Patricia's life drew to a close.

Ida

We can do no great things;
Only small things with great love.

—Mother Teresa

The occasional inheritable nature of ovarian cancer is part of the story of Ida, a Canadian who originally came from Europe. Her mother died of the disease at the age of 52. Shortly after becoming a grandmother, Ida too would contract it. After her surgery, she was feeling so good that she and her husband wanted to go back to Europe for a visit. But would she still be able to go?

I WAS BORN IN EUROPE AND MOVED to Canada when I was a teenager. My husband is also from Europe. Last year we went home to Europe for three weeks. My daughter is in nursing. My son is married and lives with a three-year-old son. My husband and I love to babysit our grandson.

My husband is retired, and I retired when I was diagnosed with the disease. I was sorry to have to leave my job. I was working at making conveyor systems for the automotive industry. There is big money in that business. When our children were small I stayed home and worked part time. Then when they were in school full time I went to work at the conveyor company. I have a good relationship with the company staff, and they still invite me to the Christmas dinner.

Intermittent Bleeding

I was diagnosed a couple of years ago in the winter. I had been having trouble with intermittent bleeding for two to three years, and I got an ultrasound every six months. I was seeing a gynecologist. I had another ultrasound in the fall of 2000, and my family doctor called me (not my gynecologist) and said, "I see something on the ultrasound; we would like to check it out a little more and see exactly what it is."

He said we would schedule a scan, but it will take a while because it is so backed up. It took until after Christmas. My family doctor said that it might be cancerous, so you'd better go and see your gynecologist right away. I went and saw him, and he still didn't know because he hadn't looked at the pictures. He said that we would have another scan in six months, and I said that I thought he had better look at the pictures from the scan right away.

So he did and then he gave me an internal exam and felt the mass right away. It was seven centimetres long, and then they were scheduling the CA-125 [blood test that shows the level of antigen in the blood known to mark tumours] and X-rays, and I had already had the X-rays. They were telling me this would take a week and that would take a week, and I told them I don't have that much time! I said it will have to be faster than that, so I arranged it myself and got in the next day. Of course the CA-125 was over 1000—normal is 35. I was diagnosed at stage three. It is terribly hard to diagnose this type of cancer.

My daughter was terribly worried because my mother had ovarian cancer; she died when she was 52. So my mother died of ovarian cancer and now I have ovarian cancer, and my daughter was terribly worried. I said that maybe she could have some tests done, and sure enough the cancer centre provided us with some tests that were covered by OHIP [Ontario Health Insurance Plan]. She just got her results back a couple of days before Christmas and they were negative. She said that was the nicest present she had ever received. She had the BRCA [breast cancer gene] test, which has been approved and is 95 percent accurate.

I was referred to a gynecologic oncologist within seven days, and I had the surgery within another week. Altogether it was two weeks from diagnosis to surgery. I was happy with that. I had the surgery and I felt much better after that, and then I was on chemo for six months. When I had finished the chemo my CA-125 was down to 17.

Plans to Travel

So then we made arrangements to go to Europe right away, because I was feeling so good and things were going in the right direction. Then when we came back in November I had another checkup and CA-125 was already back up to around 300. So we let it go for a while, and then I went back on chemo in the New Year and it did come down somewhat again.

I have all the CA-125s written down somewhere; I can't remember them offhand. I just sort of managed with the way things were. I wasn't in any pain and I wasn't uncomfortable, and then in the summer last year, all of a sudden my bowel movements stopped. So I had a bowel obstruction in the beginning of September. The gynecologic oncologist did another surgery and said that the abdomen was quite full with cancer and she couldn't get it all, but she got what she could. And then she gave me a colostomy, which is working fine, and she also put me on a study drug. This one doesn't even have a name yet, just a number: it is OSI-177.

Ida died in her home 28 months after her diagnosis of ovarian cancer.

Martha

Be glad of life, for it gives us a chance to love and to work and to play,
And to look at the stars.

—from "Footpath to Peace," by Henry van Dyke

After 43 years of marriage and raising three girls, Martha knows the value of family. And after she was diagnosed with ovarian cancer, besides praying that her girls would never get it, she prayed that it wouldn't devastate her family. "There was a time when I thought that I should run away and hide, and then they wouldn't have to worry about me," she said. "One does have these funny, flitting ideas." But she's managed to cope with such fears and others, because, in the end, when it comes to worry, she asks, "What difference does it make?"

I AM 65 YEARS OLD, AND I've been married for almost half a century to the same man. My husband and I are second cousins, because my father and his mother were first cousins. Our grandfathers were brothers. We have three girls between the ages of 36 and 41 years. I'm also a grandmother. I'll see the youngest one, who is four months old.

No one else in my family has had ovarian cancer, but my middle daughter thought I should go for genetic testing. My gynecologic oncologist agreed, and we found out that there were some incidents of cancer in my extended family, of breast cancer, for example. Also, my mother died of cancer, but she was a lifelong smoker. She developed lung cancer when she was 73, and it metastasized to the brain. It was not guaranteed that she would get cancer, but the chances were high that would happen; it wasn't a surprise. Then last December my sister was diagnosed with breast cancer. That was a real shock! My sister is eight years younger than I. That was highly unexpected.

I know that the genetic tests are not foolproof, but they did show that I don't carry a gene that could be passed on to my children. If my children are concerned, they can go for testing on their own. It is covered apparently by OHIP in Ontario, but in B.C. it isn't. Our middle daughter said that when my sister developed breast cancer, it improved her chance for contracting something. I just hope and pray that my girls don't get cancer. It doesn't seem to be predictable. So cancer is in my family, but ovarian cancer isn't; it just appeared out of the blue.

Doctors and Diagnosis

I was diagnosed two years ago. In February, almost two and a half years ago, I had a pap smear and there was nothing. Everything was quite normal. In June I started to feel uncomfortable, and I thought that I had a bladder infection. I'd had one before. It was a long time ago, but I remember you feel kind of urgent, and things weren't right. So I made an appointment to see my family doctor, but she was away. There was another doctor who saw me, and I explained that I had this feeling of things not being quite right. Earlier I had sharp pains across the abdomen, and I had no idea what it was because it disappeared within 20 minutes. When I called the doctor it was lunchtime, and by the time lunch was over it had disappeared.

Then it reoccurred one more time. When I mentioned that to the doctor, he ordered an ultrasound. After I had the ultrasound and got a clear message that everything was fine, I realized that the ultrasound only looked at the upper abdomen. I made another appointment because I still wasn't feeling right. The next report said that everything was great. So I made another appointment, and again my doctor was away. The other doctor was there, and he was defensive. He looked at me and he said, "I didn't want to see you again. Go and see your own family doctor."

So I went to the desk and I said, "I have to see my family doctor. I have to see her because this man doesn't want to." It was just after the long weekend in July, which is a four-day week, and she was only working two days, but they squeezed me in. She immediately sent me for an ultrasound of the lower abdomen. And I knew from the expression on the technician's face that the results were not good. My family doctor called me right after she got the results of the ultrasound and said that she was moving heaven and earth to get me into the hospital. And she did. She and the oncologist, they just burned up the ground.

Once my family doctor realized there was a problem, I had excellent medical care. She referred me to the oncologist, who was able to see me right away, within a week. This is as I remember it. Perhaps it was more spread out, but within a few days or a week. I had the operation quickly, which was wonderful because I didn't have time to panic. I just had a lot of work to do because I was going to be off for six months. Fortunately, it was summertime, so I had finished most of my work, and summer is tidy-up time. I just worked and worked and worked until I got things to where I felt that I could leave them, and then headed off. It was a wonderful distraction. So I was very happy about that.

Then, within two and a half weeks of the operation, they started chemo. There was no delay—it was just fantastic. I was very lucky. With my sister it was the same way: she saw an oncologist very quickly after her family doctor determined that there was a problem. I went with her to see the gynecologic oncologist, the week before Christmas. And she had chemo that week. She was given the option to wait until after Christmas, and she said no. The doctors have been excellent.

My family doctor felt awful because every time I saw her, I asked her whether I should stay on hormone replacement therapy. Well, she would weigh up the possibilities, and she said it would probably help prevent osteoporosis, so I should stay on it. When I saw her after my diagnosis, she was castigating herself for insisting that I carry on. I don't think that there is any link between the HRT and ovarian cancer, but I think that she thought that she was misadvising me. She really doesn't need to feel badly about that. HRT has got some bad press.

Telling Everyone

After seeing the oncologist, I went back to work and spoke to my supervisor to let her know. We are good friends, and I wanted to let her know. My husband knew right at the outset. He's very pragmatic. He deals with things as they happen; he doesn't get excited. I think only twice I have known him to swear. He's very gentle and accepting. I phoned my children as soon as I got home that evening—one was out West—and that was on a Thursday. On the Sunday we were at a potluck supper with old friends and I didn't say anything. The next day at work, I worked Monday and Tuesday, and then Wednesday I had to stay home and go through the scrubbing out process before the operation on Thursday.

So on Monday I sent an email to everyone on my address list just to let them know that I wouldn't be around for six months. The result of this was totally unexpected; I never even thought about what people would do. But the word spread all over my workplace because I know a lot of people there, and over the next few weeks there was a deluge of cards, letters, calls, emails, and flowers. I was flabbergasted! I didn't say much in the email—I just said that I was having an operation, followed by chemotherapy. I just couldn't bring myself to say more, but I did tell my children what it was. I didn't realize that I had that many friends. It gave me something to do, to write thank-you cards.

It wasn't really a question of coping—you just deal with it, and it's there. One of the best things was that the cancer centre advised me to see a social worker fairly early on, and the reason was that I was having trouble sleeping; I was taking Ativan at night. And sometimes during the day, chemo made me frantic and quite jumpy so they advised me to see a social worker. Privately I thought, what for? But they teamed me up with a social worker, and she just let me talk.

She also pointed out that I wasn't dying. There were two things I could do. I could curl up and not talk to anyone, or just get on with it, and my natural inclination is to get on with it. I made myself a promise that I would try not to upset everyone else. I have not done that and I don't plan to because I know from experience with other people that it is hard to deal with. I've managed so far. No, I don't think you would succumb. But you wonder when you are on the other side of this invisible barrier. When it comes down to it, what else can you do? Well, you lose control of your life for a period, and you can regain it up to a point.

I have to tell you that I haven't read up on this disease. If it was something like arthritis or something, I would. But with this one I haven't. I asked only the questions that I need the answers for. My oncologist respects that and doesn't deluge me with stuff I don't want to know. That's another way I deal with it: taking it in little bits, rather than suddenly being faced with the overall picture.

I know what the end is, and I have been thinking about that a lot and coming to terms with it. I get a lot of support from my church and from singing in the choir. I question my faith on occasion, but it has given me a lot of support in the middle of the night when things get icky. How will I deal with things down the road? I don't know. You can't tell. The main thing is trying to keep this from devastating my family. There are ways of dying that are less agonizing than others for other people. I really don't want to devastate them. There was a time when I thought that I should run away and hide, and then they wouldn't have to worry about me. One does have these funny, flitting ideas.

The Operation and Chemo

The operation was on the Thursday, and within a few days my husband had to go to Europe for a conference. My daughters got organized by email, and they took turns being with me until he got back, which was incredible. So our nursing daughter from up north came down, and she took me to the hospital on the morning of the operation and then my husband joined her. Our daughter who lives west of the city came in after the operation for a visit, and then my other daughter came back and brought her children. Then my other daughters came back and stayed here between packing up their house and moving out West. It all worked out beautifully because one arrived before the others had to leave.

By that time I was starting chemo. My daughter dropped me off at the hospital. My other daughter, fortunately, came down to the hospital and arrived just as I reacted very badly to the Taxol chemical. I was grateful that she was there because I was kind of whacked. She was there when they tried a slower drip that didn't work. And I was very happy that she was there. The next day my third daughter had to fly west, and my other daughter was here with the kids. She stayed until my husband got back. So it was just fantastic, because she had to come 600 kilometres. And my daughter from up north came. It was just amazing what my three daughters managed to do. That was a huge support. Friends dropped in and brought things to eat. There were just so many people who were thinking of me and praying for me; I was on prayer lists as far away as Australia.

I worked out a system with the church and with the choir. I love singing. I said I would keep going except in the rather fragile periods after chemotherapy where you avoid infection. I was not ill from the chemo, and I was not fatigued; I didn't have any side effects apart from the initial allergy to the Taxol. The only problem was that my white cell count went down in the middle so that for several weeks I couldn't have chemo. They switched from Taxol to something I can't remember and mixed it with carboplatin, about this time when the white cells were being uncooperative. The oncologist read a paper about a study that said that carboplatin on its own was just as effective as carboplatin with the other stuff. And in view of the effects she suggested that we try just the carbo, and lo and behold, I was able to finish the last few treatments.

I went back to work in January, and I felt like a sham because I felt fine most of the time once I recovered. The operation did kind of lay me out and I lost a lot of weight. I didn't lose or gain anything before then; there was no change to my weight at all. I felt that I was bloated, but I thought I had picked up something, a bug. I went right back to work. The first day was a little tough, and my workload had been rearranged a little bit. Somebody filled in for me when I was off. Some of the things that had been offloaded onto a colleague who had had breast cancer 10 years before insisted that I didn't take it back, although I wanted them, because I liked what I was doing. But our workloads had been out of balance over the years for various reasons. It turned out to be a good rearrangement: we were running a very difficult student appeal and it was very stressful.

So I worked from January to June, then I retired partly because I wanted to and partly because I knew that the odds were good that I would get another bout of this, and I really didn't want to go through that whole process of getting people scrambling to fill in for me. So I called it quits, and so did two other colleagues at the same time, which left only one secretary. That was pretty rough. The whole office was being revamped.

Recurrence

I have had one recurrence. I was fine at my May appointment. The blood counts were fine, but the oncologist called a few days after the August appointment and said that the CA-125 count was up to over 100, and it had been down to about 12 to 14. So she sent me for a CT scan, which was scheduled for September. I knew that there must be a problem, but I decided that I would do what I had planned to do anyway. So I went up north, where one of my daughters had arranged a swim for the cure based on one that has run on the Severn River for the last several years.

She always swam in the Severn River, but she decided last year she would do one of her own, largely because of what happened to me. And so she did, and I had collected lots of sponsors and went ahead with it. Her son, our grandson, raised more money than anyone else, and he just turned 12. He did a super job, not because he intended to, but his mom told him to alert the cottagers along the four-kilometre stretch of river where the swim was passing just to let them know if they wanted to wave and shout hurray at the swimmers. I guess one of the people offered to sponsor him. Eventually he raised over $700. For a child who isn't out-going, I thought that was quite fantastic. So anyway, I swallowed a lot of river water. It was very rough!

I practised in the local pool, and I am doing it again this summer. Forty lengths is one kilometre, and I worked up to fifty lengths. Even though I can only do less than one kilometre of the swim, my daughter has broken it up into pieces, so if you know that you can swim four and a half kilometres you start at one end, and there's a two-and-a-half-kilo-metre stretch at some other beach, and from the dock to the finishing beach is just under a kilometre. I did the last part. It's very relaxing. I went on Tuesday and swam twenty-two lengths. But then I thought I'd better stop because I didn't know what the after-effect would be. I know when I garden and dig and weed and heavy stuff I really feel it—it's mostly my legs. And I did develop stomach cramps and diarrhea.

Thinking it was the water, I went to my family doctor, and she tested for parasites and there was nothing, so I guessed it was probably the can-cer. But at that point I really didn't know. After the summer CT scan, the oncologist called and explained that I had to go through the chemo again, and since the carboplatin had worked so well the last time, she suggested that we do it again. That was fine, because it didn't cause all the awful side effects that some people get. We started in the fall, and she also had a clinical trial where you take one pill daily with the regular chemo for six sessions and see what happens. I am still on it. Although I finished the chemo at the end of January, I still take the pill. I finished the last intravenous stuff.

As a part of this study, I have to see the oncologist every three weeks and have a CT scan every six weeks, so they are keeping close tabs on me. It means I am a little tied. I'm afraid to plan ahead even two months. My husband wants to go to Stratford, and I don't dare book tickets now. But that may be stupid. We did go and see two plays in May, but there are three more that I would like to see and that means staying overnight. I am just going to wait until the next scan, which is in two weeks. If the scan is clear, I am okay to plan for the next six weeks or so. When I saw the oncologist three weeks ago, I asked if it was reasonable to book a ticket out West. Now I plan to fly the day that I next see her. If the news is bad, I'm still going, because what difference does it make?

Martha is living with recurrent ovarian cancer.

Cheryl

Circumstances may appear to wreck our lives and God's plans,
but God is not helpless among the ruins.

—Eric Liddell, Olympian

While working in a mission hospital in Brazil, Cheryl found the biggest thrill was delivering children. Bringing new life to the world. But after 15 years there, one fateful day she made her bed, folded her memories, and left. She thought she would be gone for a month. More than a year later, the 46-year-old was left dealing with her own mortality, learning how to "fight for all you're worth" and at the same, in the words of a friend, "let God be God."

I AM A NURSE, TRAINED AT a local college. After I graduated from nursing school I couldn't find a job, and I felt that God wanted me in something full time. I had also gone to Bible school in Ontario for four years and got a degree with a Bible major and missions minor. So when I heard about a mission hospital on the Amazon from another Canadian nurse who was down there, I went to Sao Paulo, in Brazil, and learned the language. From there, I moved down by the Amazon River. I started to work in a small mission hospital about 15 years ago.

I loved it, being at the mission, and that's been one of the hardest things about this year, about finding out. I think it will be a little while before I get to go back. The mission is called the Association of Baptists for World Evangelism, out of Harrisburg, Virginia. The Canadian head office is out of London. We have over 600 missionaries around the world. I think that there are 30 Canadians.

I found out I had cancer in May 2002. There is no ovarian cancer in my family, although there are other types of cancer. In fact, I had the genetic testing and it is not genetic with me. I qualified for the genetic testing because I have serous type of ovarian cancer. Even though there was no one else in the family that had it, I felt that I wanted to do it for my sister and nieces. In fact, I had not heard much about ovarian cancer at all. You hear about breast cancer all the time, but you never hear about ovarian cancer.

Fighting

Until you actually hear those words, that you have cancer, you think that it will never happen to you. I mean, I hear about people having cancer all the time, but to hear the words "you have cancer"—there is nothing to describe it. There really isn't. You just say, "Okay, now what do we do next?" And you fight for all you are worth.

At the beginning I had a complete hysterectomy and omentectomy. They removed everything they could. They got me in fast: I found out on Wednesday and had surgery the following Tuesday. Then I had massive complications after my surgery. I had a bowel obstruction and then I got septic. I was in the hospital two weeks after my surgery and in ICU for five days. As the oncologist said, "You know why this is happening to you? It's because you are a nurse." If anything could go wrong, it went wrong; it was not a great experience for me. But I didn't have a lot of pain. I was uncomfortable, but as far as pain, I didn't have any. A friend called yesterday and said, "Do you have any pain?" And I said, "No. That is one thing I do not have is pain, which is wonderful."

I had some pain today because I had this port put in yesterday for the chemo. They usually put it in your chest. My veins are basically shot. When I last had chemo, they said my veins are very fragile, so they suggested a port. Last year I had a PICC line, which is a tube hanging out of your arm. I didn't want that again. It was a pain because it is always hanging there, and I had to change the dressing every day. But the port is under the skin. Once the incision is done it heals and you won't know it's there; there will be a lump there, but you can take a shower. Well, I did have a shower, but I don't know if I was supposed to or not. I just had to be very careful, that's all..

I finished my first round of chemo in December last year and then was clear. The chemo worked, because when I had my CT scan in December, they said that there was no evidence of disease. Then in April my CA-125 was 15 (well below normal). When I went in July, the oncologist found something on my exam and my CA-125 was over 1400. It went very quickly. It is very progressive. I haven't been back to the mission since then. My mission doctor wouldn't let me go back; he thought that I at least should stay here for this year. So I was working toward that, and I was hoping to be clear at every three-month checkup and then go back at the beginning of next year, but that has of course changed.

So, I am in the middle of chemo right now. I just had one and there are five more treatments to go. It's a clinical trial with carboplatin and OSI-774; it is a pill that I take. You see the carboplatin worked before; it shrunk the tumour before, so the oncologist is trying that again along with the OSI-774.

The cancer is spread all over; it isn't in any specific place. It's all over in my omentum and my lymph nodes. I hadn't been feeling real well the last few months, but I also was having gallstones. Gallstones had shown up in my previous CAT scans, so I had gone to my family doctor and I thought I was having problems with my gallbladder. So he referred me to a surgeon and I was booked for surgery, actually next week. However, when I went to see the oncologist in July, she said that the problems are probably from the cancer and not from the gallbladder. I have had constant nausea and some pain, and just vomiting and stuff, and she feels that it is the cancer. So, my gallstone surgery was cancelled.

Faith and Fairness

Of course, my faith has been my source of strength from the very beginning. If I didn't have a relationship with the Lord, I'd be lost. I honestly and truly do not know what people do who don't have the Lord. I really don't. I know that being surrounded by a mission family means I am surrounded by prayer. I talked to my administrator yesterday, and he said that they had a meeting yesterday about something else, and they were praying for me. And I know that people literally around the world have been praying for me since the very beginning. Because of that, God has given me a real peace about this whole thing, and as a Christian I believe that God is sovereign over everything, and that he is in control over everything that happens in my life and there is a reason and purpose for this.

If I look at this as a human being, it's so hard for me to understand, because here I was working down on the Amazon River, giving my life for people there. If I look at it from a human perspective, I would say that this isn't fair, it isn't right because I was doing something for other people. But I believe that God has a purpose for this. This is what I draw on as a source of strength. I know that God is in control of this, and if it is his will for me to die of cancer then that's the way it is. My only desire is that he be glorified through this. I believe that God has a purpose and a plan for each of us, and I think that his purpose and plan for me is to have cancer at this time, and I may never know what the reason is. It is the hardest thing that I ever had to go through. I mean, it's hard to understand.

A couple of people have said to me, "You don't deserve this," and I say to them, "It has nothing to do with what I deserve. I deserve far worse than this." But when I think about it and I think about having to give up my life here, that's nothing. What I have to face for eternity is far better. I know that I am going to spend eternity in heaven with God, and that is far better than the suffering that is here on this earth. So that is what I draw on, my faith in God and my relationship with him. He is in control of what happens to me, and I don't have to worry about it. You know, I talked to another gal who has ovarian cancer and she joined a support group, but it just really isn't my thing. I have such a strong church family, and they have been very supportive. I have some wonderful friends and a great family. My sister calls me every day, and I have other friends who check on me all the time. So a support group just isn't something that appeals to me.

My family has the same faith as I do. I have a brother that doesn't share the faith, but the rest of my family does. My mom and dad are doing okay. It's been hard for them, but they trust in the Lord; that is where my example comes from. I think that it is very hard for them. You know, my mom said, "It is not like you are 80 years old—you are 46, and you have to fight this all you can. You can't sit in the corner and curl up and die, that's not the way to do it!" It has been very hard for my one sister, but at the same time she knows that God is in control of this.

It is hard just being together as a family. We were together this past weekend as a family for the first time in 10 years, and just looking at my nieces and nephews, I wonder, am I ever going to see them married and have children and stuff like that? But really, in light of eternity, things like that are not that important. Well, they are important, but only here on this earth.

One of the hardest things is that I can't go back to Brazil, but it is easier now than it would have been a year ago. If they had told me a year ago that I couldn't go back, it would have been harder because I have been gone now for one and a half years. There were so many delights there. For the last eight years I did all the deliveries at the hospital, so that was my biggest thrill. Also, establishing relationships with the girls— most of the girls were between the ages of 14 and 20, and most of them were first-time mothers. Many of them just don't have a relationship with their mothers, so I felt like I was their mother type, and I think that a lot of girls thought of me that way.

I did a prenatal clinic as well as doing the deliveries. It was good, because a lot of those girls needed advice about general life issues. That is definitely one of the highlights. I still feel very attached to the mission family down there, and I am hoping to make one more trip back to say my farewells and so on. But that will depend on how things go. My sister would go back with me.

Giving Up Control

I will never forget when last year one of our pastors came to visit with one of his interns, and the young intern, who is just in his early 20s, he prayed and he said, "Help Cheryl to let God be God." And you know that stuck with me so much because that is just what I have to do. I have to let him control what happens, because I can't control it. The only thing I can control is my attitude. I went to Bible college, and it enforced my faith. But it also helped me to realize how much I didn't know. I grew up in the church and I went off to Bible school thinking that I knew all about the Bible, but boy, I tell you, I've learned a lot more, and there is still more to learn.

I have only been living in my own place since March. I was with my parents before that. I lived on my own for years in Brazil, and I just felt that it was time to be on my own. To live with your parents when you are in your mid-40s is hard. It isn't easy for them either. When I found out my diagnosis again, they thought that I should be moving home again, but friends have encouraged me not to, and my sister says, "Don't you dare, because you need your own space." She said that there may come a time when you have to move in with them, when you don't have a choice, but she said until you have to make that decision, keep your own place.

I had my own place in Brazil, built with funds that people had donated. When I left Brazil, I left thinking that I would only be gone for a month or so. I had no idea what my diagnosis would be. So when I left Brazil, I met together with two of the Brazilian nurses who worked at the hospital, and I said that my goal was to be back by such-and-such a date because we had a team of medical people coming from the States. I said that was my goal to be back by then, so just hang on and take care of things when I am gone. I had no idea. I mean, maybe in the back of my mind I did, but I don't know.

So I left my house like I was going to be back in a month—tablecloth, bed made—and it is still sitting there. I cleaned out my fridge and freezer, but everything else is sitting there just as I left it, which is not good down there. I have been gone for 15 months, and that is another reason that I want to get back down there; I need to wrap things up and pack things away. It isn't fair to leave it for someone else, because they won't know what to do with it. Anyway, I am hoping to go back in January or February for a visit.

It is always hot down there, with 100 percent humidity. You can get a lot more done here, because the heat just zaps the energy out of you. But you learn that really quickly, and you learn to adapt to it. The first term I was there, I didn't have air conditioning, and I don't know how I survived. You need a place where you can go to be cooled off and refreshed. Otherwise you can't make it through the day. Some rooms in the hospital were air conditioned, but others were not. The patient areas weren't, because they aren't used to it. They don't even like fans. I drink tons of water and shower three to four times a day. Even then, you are wet all the time. And the missionaries, the non-natives, have more asthmatic problems, and skin problems are a big thing. Fungus is really common there. You just learn that you have to slow down when you are there, because of the heat.

No Promises for Anyone

They call ovarian cancer the silent killer. Women need to make sure that, as much as possible, they get checked. The only thing that I would say is if anybody has any doubts about symptoms, make sure they check. After I was diagnosed, I didn't go near the Internet for the first few months because all my friends did, and they said, "Cheryl you don't want to go there. It is just not something that you should be looking at right now."

So I didn't, but I have done so since. And it is rather disconcerting looking at the statistics. If you start looking at the statistics and you think the worst, then that's just no way to live. I mean, none of us have a promise of tomorrow. We could go out today and be hit by a car and killed. We don't know. You read the obituaries in the paper, and not all the people are 90 years old. None of us have that promise. The oncologist gave me my prognosis of a year, but we don't know that. Yes, the cancer to me is rather overwhelming. That has been the thing. When she said "one year," it was like "wow." But at the same time, I don't know that: I could still live for 20 years. I don't know that.

People need to be made aware that ovarian cancer is a very devastating disease, because it is so advanced by the time they find it. That is a scary thing. But I think that things have changed with cancer so much over the years. I had an aunt who died of esophageal cancer when she was 59, and that was 22 years ago. And when I thought of having cancer, she is who I thought of. And she only lasted a few months. They diagnosed her in June and she died in August. It was just very fast. She had had some problems and had gone to the doctor, but the doctor thought it was all in her head. So there was a little bit of neglect there.

But there have been so many advances in cancer treatment since then, it is not a death sentence anymore like it used to be. It isn't a pleasant thing to go through, but it is not always a death sentence.

This summer I won two round-trip tickets to London, England. I was at a conference for the mission that I am in and they donated the air passage tickets, and I really would like to go. I have always wanted to go and I have a really close friend I grew up with who I plan to take with me. It is my goal to go on that trip as well; I was going to go in October until I found out about this. But hopefully in the spring.

Cheryl did return to Brazil, where her friends and colleagues celebrated the years they worked together. Cheryl spent 32 months living with ovarian cancer.

Afterword

Mestastasizing Plots: Telling and Un-Telling the Stories of Cancer, by Kathryn Carter, Ph.D.

The whole conception of "the story," of cause and effect, the whole idea that people have a clue as to how the world works is just a piece of laughable metaphysical colonialism perpetrated upon the wild country of time.

—Lorrie Moore

I WON'T PRETEND THAT THIS was an easy assignment for an English professor who is used to stories, as we all are to some degree, that resolve in happy endings. I am accustomed to dealing with the written stories of others as just that—stories, usually committed to page, and demanding as much empathy as I am willing to give. Even though my scholarly training alerted me to another kind of reading demanded by life stories, and even though I have read diaries, biographies, and autobiographies that are very moving, I have to admit that none has affected me in quite the same way as these have. I found myself sometimes unable to read, unable to edit as I worked through these stories or recalled a poignant interview.

It has been difficult to read these stories and difficult to shape them. I also felt more than the usual burden of ethical responsibility about getting the story right because I have learned that the life stories of those living with terminal diseases are fraught with narrative challenges.

I came to realize that our expectations about stories interfere with our ability to hear the stories of cancer in all of their messiness and fragmentariness. As I worked through these stories, I recalled for courage the memory of Esther, whom I met during the summer of 2001 and whose story appears at the beginning of this book. She was a Holocaust survivor who eventually lost her fight against cancer, but she faced the end with humour and dignity and a desire to tell the stories of her life without blinking, without apology, without self-pity. She was a woman well aware

81

of the power of story, and for years she had been sharing with local high school students her memories of Auschwitz. The importance of meeting Esther was that it quickly threw into disarray the professional distance I prefer to put between myself and life stories and, more importantly, made me reflect on my assumption that the distance between me and my subjects was orderly to begin with. It made me reflect on the role of stories in our lives and wonder, along with Lorrie Moore, if stories are just something we use to colonize the wild country of time. And when it comes to unpredictable events like ovarian cancer, it becomes perhaps more difficult to pick out a single thread of narrative with its expected twists and turns of cause and effect, those underpinnings of "story" as named by Moore. How does ovarian cancer rework the plots of life stories? This project led me to wonder if other kinds of stories might emerge once we acknowledge that cause and effect may be irrelevant to this particular plot.

In one of the few articles directly addressing cancer narratives, social science researchers Cynthia Mathieson and Henderikus Stam remind us that cancer patients are "subject to this implicit schism between that which is lived and that which is narrated" in the sense that "the ill do not live in narrative as much as they live through their illness" (283). In other words, illness threatens to drown out the life story that was there previously as it takes over; illness becomes a kind of all-consuming, colonizing story. Adding to this tendency is the propensity of medical workers, with charts and clipboards, to demand a different kind of "story" or history from the patient that may have nothing to do with the story the patient wishes to tell. In the opinion of Arthur Frank, a sociologist at the University of Calgary who has written on illness and narrative, the "story" demanded by medical practitioners represents another form of colonial imposition: the medical system elicits only certain kinds of stories and demands certain kinds of subjectivity from the patients it serves. In other words, your role in the "story" that the institution of medicine demands is clearly defined by your position as patient or doctor. Illness, too, is often seen as incompatible with the kind of life story that was unfolding before cancer "interrupted." Terminal illness, in particular, pushes our life stories down pathways that few of us would have imagined; the plots of our life stories seem to become unhooked from the moorings that once tethered the story in place. "Serious illness," writes Arthur Frank, "is a loss of the 'destination and map' that previously guided the ill person's life" (1). We—patients and editors both—struggle to find ways of narrating the new plot developments.

It is especially encouraging when a doctor like Laurie Elit recognizes that storytelling is a crucial component of the lived experience of the illness (and perhaps even its outcome) and when she struggles along with us to find new ways of narrating the stories of ovarian cancer. Arthur Frank quotes scholar Rita Charon on the value of this particular kind of medical intervention when she says that physicians need "to allow [their] own injuries to increase the potency of our care of patients, to allow our personal experiences to strengthen the empathic bonds with others who suffer" (Charon xi–xii, qtd. in Frank). Frank writes elsewhere that such an approach will lead to what he calls the "remoralization" of medicine ("Between the Ride," 1). To be remoralized or, to put it another way, even rehumanized, medicine must remember the small things. Frank talks, for example, about a doctor who crouches down so that a weak patient does not have to look up; he talks about the quiet fortitude of cancer patients such as those we've met in this book. In such quiet, even mundane moments, the larger institutional project of medicine is reminded of its mission to care for human beings (in all of their complexities). The alternative is dreadful: a medical system that "has neither the time nor interest in who people are" (2). Frank concludes by stating the value of stories to this project: "stories as a form of interaction can remoralize the world" (2).

Life stories, as captured in biographies of the famous, once famous, or almost famous, tend to follow a familiar pattern: readers are usually told about the subject's childhood, then his or her education and discovery of a life partner (or failure to keep one), before moving on to the personal or professional success that brought this person to public attention in the first place. Any difficulties are glossed over or used to illustrate strength of character. For example, the promotional material for Bill Clinton's autobiography, simply entitled *My Life*, distills the essence of the life story for readers:

> We come to understand the emotional pressures of his youth—born after his father's death; caught in the dysfunctional relationship between his feisty, nurturing mother and abusive stepfather, whom he never ceased to love and whose name he took; drawn to the brilliant, compelling Hillary Rodham, whom he was determined to marry; passionately devoted, from her infancy, to their daughter Chelsea, and to the entire experience of fatherhood; slowly and painfully beginning to comprehend how his early denial of pain led him at times in to damaging patterns of behavior.

The topography of his life story is familiar to anyone who has read other examples of this genre, but it is a model of mapping a life that holds less usefulness for those living in a time of difficulty that is not yet surmounted and may never be.

Reading stories of ovarian cancer asks us to reconsider the popular assumptions we make about biographies and autobiographies, and it forcefully reminds us that the study of autobiography presents not only literary conundrums, but ethical ones. John Paul Eakin puts it best when he says that "a narrowly conceived literary approach to autobiography fail[s] to engage much of the most important work it performs in the world" (124). Reading the stories of ovarian cancer reminds readers of the ethical commitment involved in hearing someone's story, and reminds the storytellers of the terribly important work they do by simply telling their story, no matter how disorganized or chaotic it might sometimes seem.

One of the more useful texts for thinking about illness and storytelling is Arthur Frank's book *The Wounded Storyteller: Body, Illness, and Ethics*. Drawing on his personal experiences of being wounded with cancer and watching a beloved family member succumb to cancer, Frank offers a rich theory that connects illness with narrative. His theory is framed by what he sees as a necessary movement away from "passivity ... toward activity" in negotiating the experience of illness (xi). Narrative offers a way to facilitate this movement because "wounded, people may be cared for, but as storytellers, they care for others," the latter being a more active role (xii). For ovarian cancer patients, like others whose bodies insist on taking a central, dominant role in their daily lives, speaking about their experiences gives back to these wounded some measure of independence, which can mitigate what Frank terms "medical colonization" (10). Crucial to enacting anti-colonial independence from medical colonization is, in Frank's opinion, "the ethic of voice" (10). Storytelling, then, becomes a way to draw a "new map" so that this alien landscape does not overwhelm and reduce one to total dependency. Frank carefully probes the state of "being wounded" to uncover and communicate what is essential to retaining one's autonomous humanity within the experience of illness, and he finds that storytelling is a very effective vehicle.

Cancer patients, write Mathieson and Stam, are "negotiating their way through regimens of treatment, changing bodies and disrupted lives"; therefore, telling their story "takes on renewed urgency" (284). I like to think that the most radical promise of these stories is to make readers and tellers alike realize that new forms of narratives are possible—

to recognize, along with Lorrie Moore, that imposing one kind of plot on our own lives is to colonize the wild country of time. The stories of cancer patients should lead us to recognize new kinds of stories with what I'd like to call metastasizing plots. Metastasization takes place when a genetically disorganized cancer cell breaks free and becomes mobile, reconfiguring the underlying protein skeleton. Let's claim for storytelling the metaphor hidden in metastasization and its ability to name a scattered kind of storytelling, a dynamic, mobilized "un-telling" that results when a rogue cell enters and reconfigures the skeleton of the pre-existing life story. What we are offered by this rogue cell of storytelling is the possibility of seeing afresh all kinds of plots and of reconsidering the structural and generic assumptions we bring to the idea of a "life story."

So these stories are difficult, yes, in a number of ways. But these stories are vital, and the following bibliography suggests resources for those who would like to think through the process of turning their illness into story, a process that can have important beneficial effects.

Bibliography

Prepared by Geraldine Lavery

Elit, L., Charles C., Gold I., Gafni A., Farrell, A., Tedford S., Dal Bello D., Whelan T. "Women's Perceptions about Treatment Decision Making for Ovarian Cancer." *Gynaecological Oncology* 88:2 (2003): 90–95.

This article describes a qualitative study of women's role in the treatment decision-making process once they had received the initial diagnosis of ovarian cancer. Many women reported that they felt they had no say in the course of treatment and felt directed by their physician. The article argues for shared decision making.

Felman, Shoshana, and Dori Laub. *Testimony: Crises of Witnessing in Literature, Psychoanalysis, and History.* New York: Routledge, 1992.

Shoshana and Laub bring together their expertise in the fields of literary criticism and psychiatry to pose comprehensive questions concerning relationships "between narrative and history, between art and memory, [and] between speech and survival" (xiii). In a series of essays that examine various aspects of the Holocaust, they are "looking not so much for answers as for *new enabling questions*" that may inform broader contexts (xvi). A diagnosis of ovarian cancer exemplifies one such "broader context" because of its inherent and often imminent threat of death. The relationship between speech and survival may be significant in the context of ovarian cancer. In fact, other authors in this list theorize about the various conditions and mechanisms that do tie the two closely together. As Laub explains in the chapter "Bearing Witness, or the Vicissitudes of Listening," not telling one's story "serves as a perpetuation of its tyranny ... [as] events become more and more distorted in their silent retention and pervasively invade and contaminate the survivor's daily life" (79). For those diagnosed with a terminal illness, "survival" on a daily basis becomes paramount for as long as the illness allows. As a survival tool, narrating the "something that happened to me" is important indeed.

Fitch, Margaret I., and Fran Turner. *You Are Not Alone: A Guide for Canadian Women Living with Ovarian Cancer*. Toronto: National Ovarian Cancer Association, 2003.

This publication is an excellent source of information regarding the issues that women newly diagnosed with ovarian cancer and their families face. The authors have also included references to many more primary information sources, some of them accessible via the Internet. Working with multiple contributors, Fitch and Turner provide a way to learn the language of ovarian cancer, from diagnostic terms such as "grading and staging" to "peripheral neuropathy," a condition that may develop during chemotherapy. Having the tool of language is important for those facing this life-threatening disease because it facilitates discussion between the patient and medical professionals as well as between the patient and her family and friends. There is some comfort in being able to make informed choices, and to be informed means learning a new medical language.

Frank, Arthur W. *The Wounded Storyteller: Body, Illness, and Ethics*. Chicago: University of Chicago Press, 1995.
———. "Between the Ride and the Story: Illness and Remoralization." http://www .ucalgary.ca/~frank/ride/html

This article describes the depersonalization and technologization of modern medicine and its effects on patients using Weberian language of disenchantment.

Mathieson, Cynthia, and Henderikus J. Stam. "Renegotiating Identity: Cancer Narratives." *Sociology of Health and Illness* 17:3 (1995): 283–396.

The authors refuse to privilege either cancer or its narratives in their careful theoretical balancing act. They work to show on the one hand how the narratives of cancer patients are sometimes mediated by an interview process, and on the other, how endeavours in the area of psychosocial oncology have borrowed a little too much from a medical model. Psychosocial oncology represents a kind of medical colonization of storytelling in that it uses "psychiatric indices to assess the impact of the disease" (285). The authors offer a model of storytelling for cancer patients using "open-ended identity questions" (included in the article) to encourage patients to reflect on the experience of cancer. They conclude with the useful observation that "current controversies about narrative analysis in the social sciences are … an attempt to view the culture of illness from the lives of the ill rather than from the perspective of the researcher or the medical system" (302).

Miller, Nancy K. *But Enough About Me: Why We Read Other People's Lives*. New York: Colombia University Press, 2002.

Miller's book is a charming, lively, and often amusing account of her own reactions to aging, but her work has a broader, more serious agenda. She hopes that in some way it will act as "a group biography that chronicles the transformation of women's lives after the social and political upheaval of the 1960s" (xiv). She offers, in the preface, some thoughts on both autobiography and life writing, concluding that the "power of life writing" emanates from "a tension between life and text that is never fully resolved" (xiv). Expanding on that thought, Miller fields "two [theoretical] propositions." First, she maintains that the "subjects of life writing ... are as much others as ourselves," and second, that we need not identify with someone's story in order for that story to teach us valuable lessons (xv). The latter she calls "disidentification" (xvi), an approach to catharsis that discounts the need to "identify," in some parallel sense, when one reads any form of life writing.

Her fourth chapter takes a graphic, sometimes disturbing look at the aging female body. Miller illustrates the conundrum of aging as represented by some celebrated women. Miller discusses "the shock of recognition" that so many women experience when they unexpectedly encounter their own image, especially after the age of 50. For ovarian cancer patients, who must endure an acceleration of the aging process brought on by treatment regimens, the "shock of recognition" phenomenon occurs all too often and with a sometimes devastating effect. Implied in Miller's treatment of *physical* female aging is the externality of a woman's self-image—that much of what we may expect to see, but *don't* see, in those surprise reflections is made up of imposed social and cultural criteria, not our own intrinsic ideas of worth.

Roth, Diane Sims. *An Ovarian Cancer Companion*. Burnstown, ON: General Store, 2003.

Like Ryberg (see below), Roth draws on submissions from many women who have been forced to face the challenge of ovarian cancer and uses their insight to help illustrate the points she wishes to make. In addition to the anecdotal, Roth adds some instruction on basic topics, beginning with "What Is Cancer?" and continuing with information on symptoms, diagnosis, and treatment. Assisted by the anecdotes that somehow *personalize* the information given, she also tackles some salient issues, such as "Sexuality and a Partner's Response" and "Fatigue and Stress." One contributor, Trisha Tester, does her forthright best to clarify, for family and friends of cancer patients, how best to offer help when a loved one is facing a life-and-death battle. Even though she is careful to say that she speaks from only *her* point of view, what she offers would likely resonate with many others. Roth also includes a glossary of terms and two appendices that are, again, useful references. Diane Roth brings to this project her skill as a professional journalist in selecting the submitted stories and in organizing this volume of support and instruction, a project that exemplifies the proactive role that Arthur Frank sees as both healing and liberating.

Ryberg, Maureen, ed. *Warning Sighs and Whispers: True Stories That Could Save Lives.* Bloomington, IN: First Books Library, 2003.

The stories in *Warning Sighs and Whispers* are brief examples of what many of the authors on this list have theorized. Ryberg is not only editor of this anthology but also one of those who has been wounded by ovarian cancer, and she actively undertook this project with encouragement from her husband and daughters. The contributions to this volume focus on the diagnostic process and function as a collective warning to women to be both vigilant and assertive when it comes to their well-being. Frank's theories are borne out by examples of all three types of narration, "the testimonial, the angry and the modes of treatment." This book may facilitate a deeper understanding of the kinds of issues that preoccupy someone actively undergoing treatment for ovarian cancer and how that affects the way a story is told. For some, as Fuchs, in *The Text Is Myself: Women's Life Writing and Catastrophe*, points out, telling one's story about a terminal illness is a kind of "catastrophe narration" that can lead to "action, protest and survival" (31), all of which are apparent in Ryberg's collection.

Smith, Annie. *Bearing Up with Cancer*. Toronto: Second Story Press, 2004.

The foreword to Dr. Annie Smith's illness narrative, written by Dr. Barry Rosen (a gynecological oncologist), confirms that *Bearing Up with Cancer* gave him and his team "a radically different, and immensely valuable, perspective [on ovarian cancer]" (ix). Annie Smith's book is delightfully self-illustrated and the narration is forthright, laced with humour, and also deeply personal. She offers herself, in the guise of her childhood "bear," as a guide through the maze generated by repeated diagnoses of ovarian cancer and their concomitant treatment regimens. Her technique clearly illustrates Frank's theory that storytelling is a vehicle for creating a "new map" to help chart the unfamiliar terrain of serious illness. For those who have had little or no prior experience with "medical colonization" (as described by Frank), this map is especially important. Moreover, this is an optimistic book. It urges us to remember that statistics are located on a continuum that has both positive and negative extremes. Like Stephen Jay Gould, who saw cancer statistics as a challenge, Annie Smith is determined "to be on the positive side of all those numbers" (125).

Weisman, Avery D.. *The Coping Capacity: On the Nature of Being Mortal*. New York: Human Sciences Press, 1984.

Weisman's stated purpose in writing this book is to "look at how we very ordinary folks cope and fail to cope with a variety of regularly occurring threats to our integrity and survival, which I term *expectable problems*" (xii; italics in original). Expectable problems come in many varieties, according to Weisman. A common and recurring one is fatal illness. In his preface, Weisman has some interesting comments regarding the nature of cancer. He sees cancer as prototypical of fatal illness, so much so that it has become a symbol for death, a symbol that is at once both iconic and mythic. Chapter Two is devoted to a deeper analysis of cancer as an "expectable problem," and he adds that "cancer mortality has become a metaphor transcending boundaries of disease" (15–16).

Books in the Life Writing Series
Published by Wilfrid Laurier University Press

Auto/biography in Canada: Critical Directions edited by Julie Rak • 2005 / viii + 264 pp. / ISBN 0-88920-478-0

Tracing the Autobiographical edited by Marlene Kadar, Linda Warley, Jeanne Perreault, and Susanna Egan • 2005 / viii + 280 pp. / ISBN 0-88920-476-4

Must Write: Edna Staebler's Diaries edited by Christl Verduyn • 2005 / viii + 304 pp. / ISBN 0-88920-481-0

Food That Really Schmecks by Edna Staebler • 2007 / xxiv + 334 pp. / ISBN 978-0-88920-521-5

163256: A Memoir of Resistance by Michael Englishman • 2007 / xvi + 112 pp. (14 b&w photos) / ISBN 978-1-55458-009-5

The Wartime Letters of Leslie and Cecil Frost, 1915–1919 edited by R.B. Fleming • 2007 / xxxvi + 384 pp. (49 b&w photos, 5 maps) / ISBN 978-1-55458-000-2

Johanna Krause Twice Persecuted: Surviving in Nazi Germany and Communist East Germany by Carolyn Gammon and Christiane Hemker • 2007 / x + 170 pp. (58 b&w photos, 2 maps) / ISBN 978-1-55458-006-4

Watermelon Syrup: A Novel by Annie Jacobsen with Jane Finlay-Young and Di Brandt • 2007 / x + 268 pp. / ISBN 978-1-55458-005-7

Becoming My Mother's Daughter: A Story of Survival and Renewal by Erika Gottlieb • 2008 / x + 178 pp. (36 b&w illus., 17 colour) / ISBN 978-1-55458-030-9

Bearing Witness: Living with Ovarian Cancer edited by Kathryn Carter and Lauri Elit • 2009 / viii + 94 pp. / ISBN 978-1-55458-055-2